Tips and tricks for avoiding common errors on the Minimum Data Set (MDS)

by Anna May Xu

Table of contents

Overview 6
Section A: Identification information 8
A0310 = 0 (not first assessment) 8
A0310-E = 1 (first assessment) 12
A1600 (entry date) 14
A1700 (type of entry) 14
A1900 (admission date) 17
A2400 (Medicare stay) 18
Section D: Mood 22
Residents are a danger to themselves 23
Change in PHQ-9 total severity score 23
Section E: Behavior 24
E0200 (behavioral symptom) 25
E0800 (rejection of care) 26
Section F: Preferences for customary routine and activities 28
Section G: Functional status 30
G0110 (activities of daily living (ADL) assistance) 31
Rule of 3 32
Instructions for the rule of 3 34

- Rule of 3 exceptions..36
- Tips for coding section G correctly........................37
- G0400 (functional limitation in range of motion)....39

Section H: Bladder and bowel 40
- H0200 (urinary toileting program) 40
- H0100 (appliances)..42
- H0200-C (urinary toileting program or trial)...........44

Section I: Active diagnoses..46
- I2300 (urinary tract infection) 50
- Z codes (aftercare codes) 52

Section J: Health conditions 54
- J0100 (pain management) 54
- J0300 – J0600 (pain assessment interview).........58
- J1550-A (fever) 62
- J1550-C (dehydrated) 63
- J1700 (fall history on admission/entry or reentry) .64
- J1800 (falls since admission) 66
- J1900-C (number of falls with major injury)...........67

Section K: Swallowing and nutritional status 68
- K0510 (nutritional approaches)..............................69
- K0710 (percent intake by artificial route)................73

Section M: Skin conditions 74
    M0210 (unhealed pressure injuries) 74
    M0300 (current number of unhealed pressure injuries at each stage) 75
    M0300-A (stage 1 pressure injuries) 76
    M0300-B (stage 2 pressure injuries) 77
    M0300-C (stage 3 pressure injuries) 78
    M0300-D (stage 4 pressure injuries) 79

Section N: Medications 80
    N0410 (medications received) 80

Section O: Special treatments, procedures, and programs 82
    O0100-M (isolation or quarantine for active infectious disease) 82
    O0300 (pneumococcal vaccine) 86
    O0400 (therapies) 90

Section P: Restraints and alarms 94

Section V: Care area assessment (CAA) summary .. 98
    Care area assessments (CAAs) 99
    V0100 (items from the most recent prior OBRA or scheduled PPS assessment) 104

Section X: Correction request 106
- Quality Improvement Evaluation System (QIES) 106
- How to correct errors 109
- Item set code (ISC) 110

Section Z: Assessment administration 114
- Z0100 (Medicare Part A billing) 114
- Z0400 (signatures of persons completing the assessment or entry/death reporting) 116
- Z0500 (signature of RN assessment coordinator verifying assessment completion) 120

Overview

When people get admitted to a nursing home, the staff perform assessments on them to determine how much care and resources they'll need. The information from these assessments is coded into minimum data set (MDS) data. Some of the sections on the resident assessment instrument can be a bit tricky to fill out. This book will go over some common mistakes on the MDS and how to avoid them.

Tricky resident assessment sections

- **A**: Identification information
- **D**: Mood
- **E**: Behavior
- **F**: Preferences for customary routine and activities
- **G**: Functional status
- **H**: Bladder and bowel
- **I**: Active diagnoses
- **J**: Health conditions
- **K**: Swallowing and nutritional status
- **M**: Skin conditions
- **N**: Medications
- **O**: Special treatments, procedures, and programs
- **P**: Restraints and alarms
- **V**: Care area assessment (CAA) summary
- **X**: Correction request
- **Z**: Assessment administration

Section A: Identification information

The first part of a resident's assessment is their identification.

A0310. Type of Assessment		
Enter Code	**A. Federal OBRA Reason for Assessment** 01. **Admission** assessment (required by day 14) 02. **Quarterly** review assessment 03. **Annual** assessment 04. **Significant change in status** assessment 05. **Significant correction** to **prior comprehensive** assessment 06. **Significant correction** to **prior quarterly** assessment 99. **None of the above**	
Enter Code	**B. PPS Assessment** **PPS Scheduled Assessment for a Medicare Part A Stay** 01. **5-day** scheduled assessment **PPS Unscheduled Assessment for a Medicare Part A Stay** 08. **IPA** - Interim Payment Assessment **Not PPS Assessment** 99. **None of the above**	
Enter Code	**E. Is this assessment the first assessment** (OBRA, Scheduled PPS, or Discharge) **since the most recent admission/entry or reentry?** 0. **No** 1. **Yes**	
Enter Code	**F. Entry/discharge reporting** 01. **Entry** tracking record 10. **Discharge** assessment-**return not anticipated** 11. **Discharge** assessment-**return anticipated** 12. **Death in facility** tracking record 99. **None of the above**	
Enter Code	**G. Type of discharge** - Complete only if A0310F = 10 or 11 1. **Planned** 2. **Unplanned**	
Enter Code	**G1. Is this a SNF Part A Interrupted Stay?** 0. **No** 1. **Yes**	
Enter Code	**H. Is this a SNF Part A PPS Discharge Assessment?** 0. **No** 1. **Yes**	

A0310 = 0 (not first assessment)

A0310-E asks whether the assessment is the first assessment since their most recent admission, entry, or re-entry. **No = 0** and **Yes = 1**.

Enter Code	**E. Is this assessment the first assessment** (OBRA, Scheduled PPS, or Discharge) **since the most recent admission/entry or reentry?** 0. **No** 1. **Yes**

Here are the instances where you should code
A0310-E = 0.

Death of resident or entry tracking record

You should code A0310-E = 0 if either of the following occurs:

- the MDS item is only an entry tracking record (A0310-F = 01)
- the resident has died (A0310-F = 12)

If MDS entry is		Result
A0310-F = 01 (entry tracking record)	or	
A0310-F = 12 (death in the facility tracking record)	or	
		A0310-E = 0

Standalone Part A PPS discharge assessment

If a resident has a standalone Part A PPS discharge assessment, then you should code A0310-E = 0. A Part A PPS discharge assessment requires:

- A0310-A = 99 (none of the above reason for assessment)
- A0310-B = 99 (none of the above PPS assessment)
- A0310-F = 99 (none of the above entry and discharge reporting)
- A0310-H = 1 (part of a Part A PPS discharge assessment)

If MDS entry is		Result
A0310-A = 99 (none of the above reason for assessment)	and	
A0310-B = 99 (none of the above PPS assessment)	and	
A0310-F = 99 (none of the above entry and discharge reporting)	and	
A0310-H = 1 (part of a Part A PPS discharge assessment)	and	
		A0310-E = 0

Interim payment assessment

If a resident is getting an interim payment assessment, then you should code A0310-E = 0. An interim payment assessment requires:

- A0310A = 99 (none of the above reason for assessment)
- A0310B = 08 (interim payment assessment)
- A0310F = 99 (none of the above entry and discharge reporting)
- A0310H = 0 (no Part A PPS discharge assessment)

If MDS entry is		Result
A0310-A = 99 (none of the above reason for assessment)	and	
A0310B = 08 (interim payment assessment)	and	
A0310-F = 99 (none of the above entry and discharge reporting)	and	
A0310H = 0 (no Part A PPS discharge assessment)	and	
		A0310-E = 0

A0310-E = 1 (first assessment)

Nursing homes code A0310-E = 1 for the first OBRA assessment, scheduled PPS assessment, or OBRA discharge assessment that they complete and submit. This item can be confusing in circumstances in which a resident is initially admitted under a payer source other than original Medicare A, thus requiring a scheduled PPS assessment.

Original Medicare A and Medicare Advantage

If a resident is admitted under a payer source other than original Medicare A, they'll usually require a scheduled PPS assessment. That means that sometimes you'll have to code A0310-E = 1, even though the nursing home has already completed or submitted another assessment.

Medicare Advantage

Residents who are on a Medicare Advantage plan may require a non-submitted PPS assessment before their first qualifying OBRA or PPS assessment. Only the first submitted assessment after admission gets coded A0310-E = 1 (yes). For example, if a resident has a completed and submitted OBRA admission assessment, but also a completed, non-submitted 5-

Day PPS assessment, then the A0310-E is coded 1 (yes).

Returning after a hospital stay

If a nursing home resident goes to the hospital and returns within 30 days, then the nursing home doesn't need to do a new admission assessment. Additionally, if there is no significant change, Medicare Advantage may require a PPS assessment, but the nursing home should not submit it.

Switching from Medicare Advantage to original Medicare A

If a resident switches from Medicare Advantage to original Medicare A, then the PPS schedule starts over. The nursing home has to complete and submit a new PPS 5-day assessment. Thus, they would code A0310-E, even though the resident had prior assessments.

A1600 (entry date)

A1600 shows the date of the most recent admission, entry, or re-entry into a nursing home. The entry date is the date that a resident is originally admitted into a nursing facility, or the date of the most recent re-admission after a discharge, whichever is more recent. This date is not changed by a leave of absence (LOA).

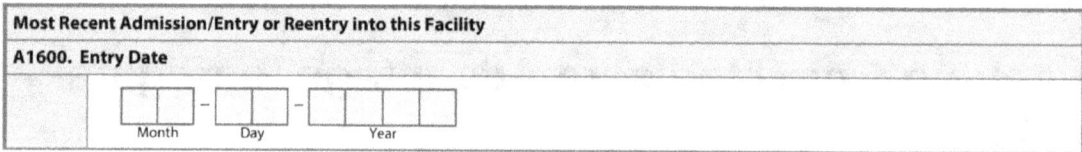

A1700 (type of entry)

A1700 shows whether the date in A1600 is an admission or reentry. This item can be coded 1 (admission) or 2 (re-entry).

A1700 = 1 (admission)

Code 1 when any one of the following occurs:

- the resident has never been admitted to the nursing home before
- the resident has been in the nursing home before, but his discharged return was not anticipated
- the resident has been in the nursing home before and his discharged return was anticipated, but he didn't return within 30 days of discharge

If the resident		Result
has never been in the nursing home before	or	
has been in the nursing home before, but the nursing home didn't think he'd return	or	
the resident has been in the nursing home before, but they thought he'd come back within 30 days and he wasn't	or	
		A1700 = 1

A1700 = 2 (re-entry)

Code 2 when all three following items occurred prior to the resident's re-entry:

- The resident was admitted to the nursing home
- The nursing home anticipated the resident's discharged return
- The resident returned to facility within 30 days of discharge

The day after the day of discharge is counted as day one when determining whether the resident returned within 30 days.

If MDS entry is		Result
A0310-A = 99 (none of the above reason for assessment)	and	
A0310B = 08 (Interim payment assessment)	and	
A0310-F = 99 (none of the above entry and discharge reporting)	and	
A0310H = 0 (no Part A PPS discharge assessment)	and	
		A1700 = 2

A1900 (admission date)

A1900 is the date that a resident's episode of care begins. This item should remain the same for all assessments in a given episode, even if the resident's care is interrupted by temporary discharges.

A1900. Admission Date (Date this episode of care in this facility began)
[__|__] - [__|__] - [__|__|__|__]
Month   Day   Year

Here are some common cases:

A resident who first goes to a nursing home will have the same A1900 (admission date) and the A1600 (entry date). His A1700 (type of admission) is 1 = admission.

A resident who goes to the hospital and then comes back will have his original A1900 date, but his A1600 will change to the most recent re-entry date. His A1700 is 2 = re-entry.

A resident who comes back after an unanticipated discharge return, or who comes back after more than 30 days at the hospital, will be considered to have a new episode of care. The nursing home will code A1900 with a new admission date.

A2400 (Medicare stay)

A2400 shows whether a resident was covered by Medicare Part A during his most recent admission or readmission. This item helps calculate short stay payment in some states. The lookback period starts at the date of A1600 (entry date) and ends at the ARD (assessment reference date).

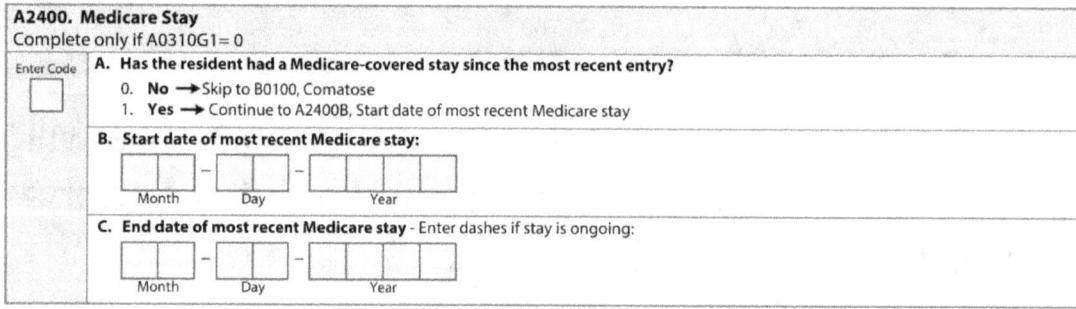

If the resident was covered by Medicare between A1600 and the ARD, then A2400-A = 1 (yes).

A2400-B is the start date of the Medicare stay. If the resident had more than one Medicare Part A stay since the A1600 date, then A2400-B is the most recent Part A stay.

A2400-C is the end date of the resident's stay. A2400-C is the day when one of the following occurred first:

- The date that the resident's benefits were exhausted, such as day 100 of the Part A stay
- The last paid day of Medicare A when the resident's payer source changes, regardless of whether the resident has moved to another bed or not
- The last day of coverage, according to the Notice of Medicare Non-Coverage (NOMNC)
- The date that the resident was discharged (A2000, discharge date)

Notes for A2400-C

If coverage doesn't end during the resident's stay: If the resident's Medicare Part A coverage will continue beyond the ARD, then enter dashes into A2400-C.

Less than 24 hospital stay: If a Medicare Part A resident goes on a therapeutic leave of absence or a hospital observation stay of less than 24 hours, without hospital admission, then this is a continuation of the Medicare Part A stay, not a new Medicare Part A stay.

Patient notification affects Medicare Part A payment and: Many people think that A2400-C is always the last day that Medicare Part A pays for the resident, or the day before the resident's discharge, but this isn't true. Even though the day of discharge isn't a paid Medicare Part A day, it is the last Medicare day, unless the resident had been informed earlier via the beneficiary notification process that covered care was going to end.

Example

Mrs. Hartmann was admitted to the nursing facility on January 15, 2021. She recovered well and the care plan team deemed her stable and able to manage her own medications and dressing changes. This meant that she was no longer qualified for Part A SNF coverage. The nursing home issued a Skilled Nursing Facility Advance Beneficiary Notice (SNFABN) and a NOMNC with the last day of coverage as January 27, 2021. Mrs. Hartmann was discharged on January 28, 2021.

Discharge assessment:

A2000 (discharge date) = 01-28-2021

A2400-A (is the stay Medicare-covered?) = 1 (yes)

A2400-B (start day of stay) = 01-15-2021

A2400-C (end date of stay) = 01-27-2021

Section D: Mood

Nursing homes attempt to do a mood interview with all residents, using either the patient health questionnaire-9 (PHQ-9) or the patient health questionnaire-9, observation version (PHQ-9-OV), which is the staff assessment. This interview is supposed to be done at time convenient for the resident, but CMS also encourages nursing homes to do the interview the day before or the day of the ARD (assessment reference date). I don't know why they want the mood interview done so close to the lookback period, but there you go.

People sometimes think that if the PHQ-9 and the clinical record don't match, then the clinical record has priority. Actually, care plans should use information from both the interview and the clinical record.

Residents are a danger to themselves

In 2019, MDS removed the coding for residents who had suicide ideation and thoughts of self-harm. However, nursing homes still must have a policy for following up with residents who say that they have thoughts of hurting himself or that they would be better off dead.

Change in PHQ-9 total severity score

Nursing homes should have a policy for when a resident has an unexpected change in their PHQ-9 total severity score. For example, the nursing home could notify the resident's physician if there is a jump of x points on the depression scale. The most important thing is that the nursing home does something to address the resident's change in mood.

Section E: Behavior

People sometimes get delusion and hallucination mixed up on the MDS.

E0100: Potential Indicators of Psychosis

E0100. Potential Indicators of Psychosis	
↓ Check all that apply	
☐	A. Hallucinations (perceptual experiences in the absence of real external sensory stimuli)
☐	B. Delusions (misconceptions or beliefs that are firmly held, contrary to reality)
☐	Z. None of the above

A **delusion** is a fixed, false belief that is (1) not shared by others and (2) the resident holds true, even in the face of evidence to the contrary. Delusions are common for residents with dementia. For example, a resident may say, "I need to pick up my three children from school. They are 6, 9, and 11 years old," and continues to hold this belief even though the staff have told her that all of her children are adults.

A **hallucination** is the perception of the presence of something that is not actually there. These perceptions can involve the auditory, visual, smell, taste, or touch senses. For example, a resident who is experiencing a hallucination may say, "I heard my children crying because I haven't picked them up from school."

E0200 (behavioral symptom)

E0200: Behavioral Symptom—Presence & Frequency

E0200. Behavioral Symptom - Presence & Frequency		
Note presence of symptoms and their frequency		
Coding: 0. Behavior not exhibited 1. Behavior of this type occurred 1 to 3 days 2. Behavior of this type occurred 4 to 6 days, but less than daily 3. Behavior of this type occurred daily	↓ Enter Codes in Boxes	
	☐	A. **Physical behavioral symptoms directed toward others** (e.g., hitting, kicking, pushing, scratching, grabbing, abusing others sexually)
	☐	B. **Verbal behavioral symptoms directed toward others** (e.g., threatening others, screaming at others, cursing at others)
	☐	C. **Other behavioral symptoms not directed toward others** (e.g., physical symptoms such as hitting or scratching self, pacing, rummaging, public sexual acts, disrobing in public, throwing or smearing food or bodily wastes, or verbal/vocal symptoms like screaming, disruptive sounds)

Residents may show new behaviors due to unrecognized needs, preferences, or illness. Staff should evaluate new behaviors and determine whether the resident can get treatment or medical intervention. E0200 shows these new behavioral symptoms that are common in residents with impaired cognition:

- physical behavioral symptoms directed toward others (E0200A)
- verbal behavioral symptoms directed toward others (E0200B)
- other behavioral symptoms not directed toward others (E0200C)
- rejection of care (E0800)
- wandering (E0900)

E0800 (rejection of care)

E0800: Rejection of Care—Presence & Frequency

E0800. Rejection of Care - Presence & Frequency	
Enter Code	Did the resident reject evaluation or care (e.g., bloodwork, taking medications, ADL assistance) that is necessary to achieve the resident's goals for health and well-being? Do not include behaviors that have already been addressed (e.g., by discussion or care planning with the resident or family), and determined to be consistent with resident values, preferences, or goals. 0. Behavior not exhibited 1. Behavior of this type occurred 1 to 3 days 2. Behavior of this type occurred 4 to 6 days, but less than daily 3. Behavior of this type occurred daily

Rejection of care is behavior that interrupts or interferes with the delivery or receipt of care.

Cognitively impaired residents' right of refusal

When a cognitively impaired resident can't talk or voice their desires, it can be difficult to determine whether they're rejecting care or exercising their right of resident choice. They can show physical aversion to care or verbal declines. However, such behaviors aren't automatically considered rejection of care. In these cases, the nursing home staff should ask the resident's family about their values, preferences, and goals.

Rejection of care in the care plan

Rejection of care is coded as rejection of care, even if the rejection of care is included in the care plan. Be sure that the rejection occurred during the 7-day lookback period and the rejection is considered a rejection of the resident's own goals for himself.

Coding all behaviors

It's important to document all behaviors, even if they occur daily as part a chronic disease or are part of a care plan.

Section F: Preferences for customary routine and activities

Section F is the only section where input from family and relatives should be coded. If a resident is rarely or never understood, the assessor should ask their family what the resident's preferences are. If the resident doesn't have family, then the assessor uses the staff assessment. All of this information should be coded in section F.

After getting the information from the resident, resident's family, or assessor, the interdisciplinary team should include this information in the resident's care plan.

F0400. Interview for Daily Preferences

Show resident the response options and say: *"While you are in this facility..."*

Coding:
1. **Very important**
2. **Somewhat important**
3. **Not very important**
4. **Not important at all**
5. **Important, but can't do or no choice**
9. **No response or non-responsive**

↓ Enter Codes in Boxes

☐	A. how important is it to you to **choose what clothes to wear**?
☐	B. how important is it to you to **take care of your personal belongings or things**?
☐	C. how important is it to you to **choose between a tub bath, shower, bed bath, or sponge bath**?
☐	D. how important is it to you to **have snacks available between meals**?
☐	E. how important is it to you to **choose your own bedtime**?
☐	F. how important is it to you to **have your family or a close friend involved in discussions about your care**?
☐	G. how important is it to you to **be able to use the phone in private**?
☐	H. how important is it to you to **have a place to lock your things to keep them safe**?

F0500. Interview for Activity Preferences

Show resident the response options and say: *"While you are in this facility..."*

Coding:
1. **Very important**
2. **Somewhat important**
3. **Not very important**
4. **Not important at all**
5. **Important, but can't do or no choice**
9. **No response or non-responsive**

↓ Enter Codes in Boxes

☐	A. how important is it to you to **have books, newspapers, and magazines to read**?
☐	B. how important is it to you to **listen to music you like**?
☐	C. how important is it to you to **be around animals such as pets**?
☐	D. how important is it to you to **keep up with the news**?
☐	E. how important is it to you to **do things with groups of people**?
☐	F. how important is it to you to **do your favorite activities**?
☐	G. how important is it to you to **go outside to get fresh air when the weather is good**?
☐	H. how important is it to you to **participate in religious services or practices**?

F0600. Daily and Activity Preferences Primary Respondent

Enter Code: ☐

Indicate primary respondent for Daily and Activity Preferences (F0400 and F0500)
1. **Resident**
2. **Family or significant other** (close friend or other representative)
9. **Interview could not be completed** by resident or family/significant other ("No response" to 3 or more items")

Section G: Functional status

Section G is one of the hardest sections to code in the MDS.

G0110: Activities of Daily Living (ADL) Assistance

G0110. Activities of Daily Living (ADL) Assistance
Refer to the ADL flow chart in the RAI manual to facilitate accurate coding

Instructions for Rule of 3
- When an activity occurs three times at any one given level, code that level.
- When an activity occurs three times at multiple levels, code the most dependent, exceptions are total dependence (4), activity must require full assist every time, and activity did not occur (8), activity must not have occurred at all. Example, three times extensive assistance (3) and three times limited assistance (2), code extensive assistance (3).
- When an activity occurs at various levels, but not three times at any given level, apply the following:
  - When there is a combination of full staff performance, and extensive assistance, code extensive assistance.
  - When there is a combination of full staff performance, weight bearing assistance and/or non-weight bearing assistance code limited assistance (2).

If none of the above are met, code supervision.

1. ADL Self-Performance
Code for **resident's performance** over all shifts - not including setup. If the ADL activity occurred 3 or more times at various levels of assistance, code the most dependent - except for total dependence, which requires full staff performance every time

Coding:
Activity Occurred 3 or More Times
0. **Independent** - no help or staff oversight at any time
1. **Supervision** - oversight, encouragement or cueing
2. **Limited assistance** - resident highly involved in activity; staff provide guided maneuvering of limbs or other non-weight-bearing assistance
3. **Extensive assistance** - resident involved in activity, staff provide weight-bearing support
4. **Total dependence** - full staff performance every time during entire 7-day period

Activity Occurred 2 or Fewer Times
7. **Activity occurred only once or twice** - activity did occur but only once or twice
8. **Activity did not occur** - activity did not occur or family and/or non-facility staff provided care 100% of the time for that activity over the entire 7-day period

2. ADL Support Provided
Code for **most support provided** over all shifts; code regardless of resident's self-performance classification

Coding:
0. **No** setup or physical help from staff
1. **Setup** help only
2. **One** person physical assist
3. **Two+** persons physical assist
8. ADL activity itself **did not occur** or family and/or non-facility staff provided care 100% of the time for that activity over the entire 7-day period

	1. Self-Performance	2. Support
A. **Bed mobility** - how resident moves to and from lying position, turns side to side, and positions body while in bed or alternate sleep furniture	☐	☐
B. **Transfer** - how resident moves between surfaces including to or from: bed, chair, wheelchair, standing position (**excludes** to/from bath/toilet)	☐	☐
C. **Walk in room** - how resident walks between locations in his/her room	☐	☐
D. **Walk in corridor** - how resident walks in corridor on unit	☐	☐
E. **Locomotion on unit** - how resident moves between locations in his/her room and adjacent corridor on same floor. If in wheelchair, self-sufficiency once in chair	☐	☐
F. **Locomotion off unit** - how resident moves to and returns from off-unit locations (e.g., areas set aside for dining, activities or treatments). **If facility has only one floor**, how resident moves to and from distant areas on the floor. If in wheelchair, self-sufficiency once in chair	☐	☐
G. **Dressing** - how resident puts on, fastens and takes off all items of clothing, including donning/removing a prosthesis or TED hose. Dressing includes putting on and changing pajamas and housedresses	☐	☐
H. **Eating** - how resident eats and drinks, regardless of skill. Do not include eating/drinking during medication pass. Includes intake of nourishment by other means (e.g., tube feeding, total parenteral nutrition, IV fluids administered for nutrition or hydration)	☐	☐
I. **Toilet use** - how resident uses the toilet room, commode, bedpan, or urinal; transfers on/off toilet; cleanses self after elimination; changes pad; manages ostomy or catheter; and adjusts clothes. Do not include emptying of bedpan, urinal, bedside commode, catheter bag or ostomy bag	☐	☐
J. **Personal hygiene** - how resident maintains personal hygiene, including combing hair, brushing teeth, shaving, applying makeup, washing/drying face and hands (**excludes** baths and showers)	☐	☐

G0110 (activities of daily living (ADL) assistance)

Activities of daily living (ADLs) are self-care activities, such as walking around, toileting, and brushing teeth. G0110 measures a resident's ability to complete their own tasks (column 1, self-performance) and the amount of nursing home staff intervention needed to complete those tasks (column 2, support).

In this section, staff only includes direct employees and facility-contracted employees, such as rehabilitation staff and nursing agency staff. It doesn't include people hired outside of the facility management, such as hospice staff, nursing students, private caretakers, or family members.

Rule of 3

All self-performance of activities of daily living code has to follow a three-step process called the "rule of 3." The following information is required for applying the rule of 3:

- an ADL activity
- how many times the resident performed the ADL activity in the 7-day lookback period
- how much staff support the resident needed for the ADL activity in the 7-day lookback period

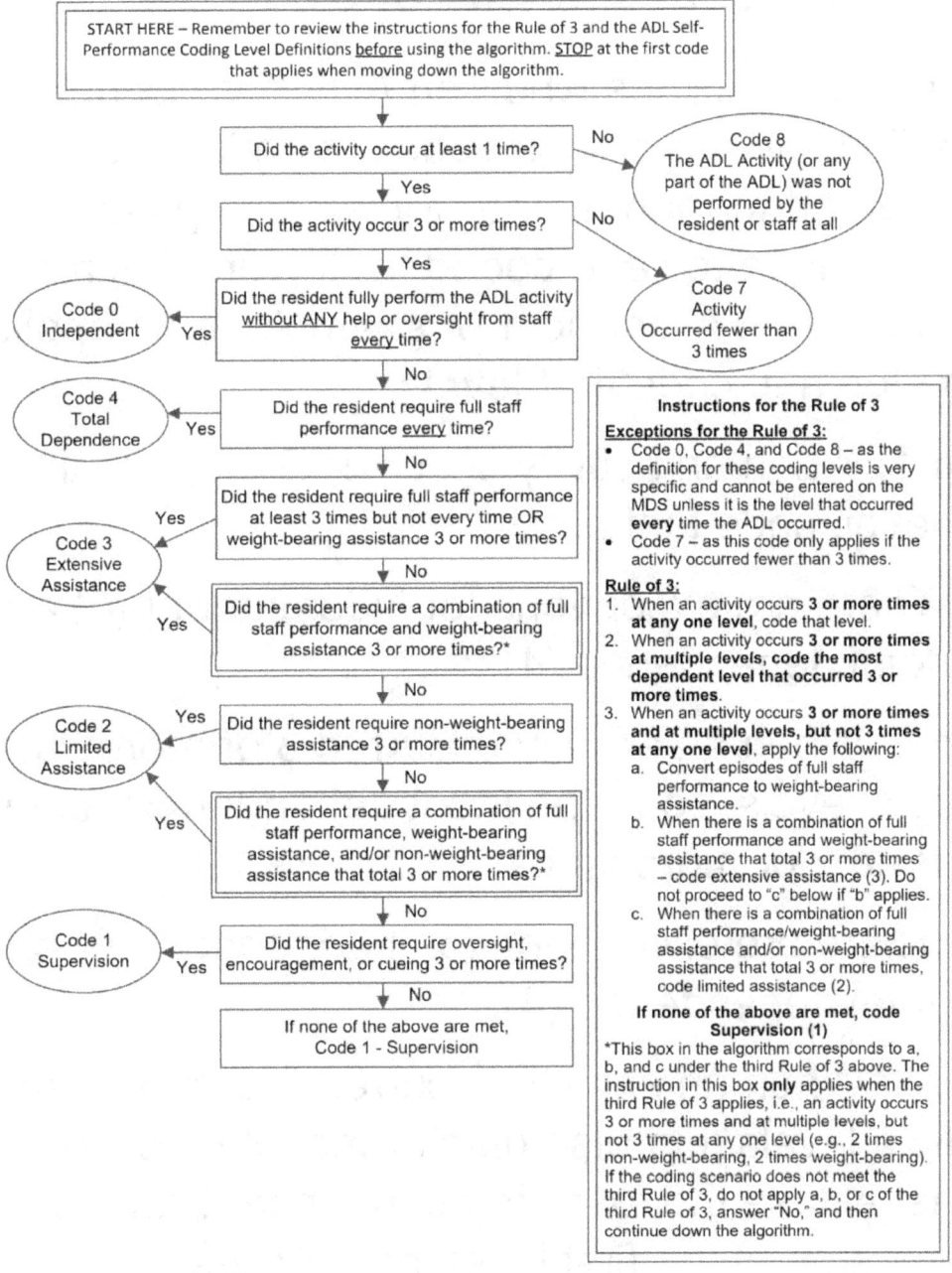

Instructions for the rule of 3

The rule of 3 applies when an ADL has occurred 3 or more times in a 7-day lookback period. In column 1, ADL self-performance, the following steps must be used in sequence and coded for the first instruction that meets the scenario. For example, if #1 applies, then stop and code that level.

Step 1: When an activity occurred 3 or more times at one level, code that level.

> There are exceptions for independent (0) and total dependence (4).

Step 2: When an activity occurred 3 or more times at multiple levels, code the most dependent level that occurred 3 or more times.

> There are exceptions for independent (0) and total dependence (4).

Step 3: When an activity occurred 3 or more times at multiple levels, but also didn't reach 3 times at any one level, use the following sequence. Same as before, stop at the first level that applies.

> **Step 3a**: If the full staff performance instances didn't occur every time an ADL was performed,

then convert those full staff performance instances to weight-bearing assistance instances. Then you can code 3 (extensive assistance).

> **Note**: You can only code 4 (total dependence) only if every single instance is a full staff performance.

Step 3b: If the resident needed full staff performance and weight-bearing assistance 3 or more times, then code 3 (extensive assistance).

Step 3c: If there is a combination of full staff performance/weight-bearing assistance, and/or non-weight-bearing assistance that total three or more times, then code 2 (limited assistance).

If none of the above apply, then code 1 (supervision).

Rule of 3 exceptions

The following ADL self-performance coding levels are exceptions to the rule of 3:

- Code 0 (independent): The ADL activity occurred at least 3 times and the resident completed their ADL activity with no help or oversight, every single time. The lookback period is 7 days.
- Code 4 (total dependence): The ADL activity occurred at least 3 times and the resident required full staff performance of that ADL activity, every single time. The lookback period is 7 days.
- Code 7 (activity occurred only once or twice): The ADL activity occurred fewer than 3 times in the 7-day lookback period.
- Code 8, (activity did not occur): The ADL activity did not occur or non-facility staff or family provided care 100% of the time for that activity over the entire 7-day lookback period.

Tips for coding section G correctly

Here are some tips for completing the MDS correctly.

Follow the definitions of the ADL activities literally

Every ADL has a list of components that define it. Only those aspects can be considered when coding the activity. This can be tricky when multiple activities from various ADLs occur simultaneously. For example, G0110A is bed mobility and consists of:

- moving to and from a lying position
- moving from side to side
- changing position while in bed or alternate sleep furniture

A resident may turn from side to side in bed during incontinence care. Even though the ADL happens during the toileting program, it should be coded under bed mobility because it matches the definition of bed mobility.

Code the resident's actual performance

Sometimes people code what they think the resident is capable of or what they should be doing, instead of what the resident actually does.

MDS must match the documentation in the clinical records

When the auditor comes, they'll check that the MDS that is coded matches the resident's clinical record. Nursing home administration should make sure that their MDS staff know how to read a chart and code accurately.

Record all instances of activities

The rule of 3 is based on how often a resident performs a particular activity of daily living. If charting is only done once per shift, it may not reflect how many times the resident performed the activity or how many times he needed help with that activity. Auditors also check for once-per-shift charting.

G0400 (functional limitation in range of motion)

Lookback period: 7 days

G0400. Functional Limitation in Range of Motion	
Code for limitation that interfered with daily functions or placed resident at risk of injury	Enter Codes in Boxes
Coding: 0. No impairment 1. Impairment on one side 2. Impairment on both sides	☐ A. Upper extremity (shoulder, elbow, wrist, hand) ☐ B. Lower extremity (hip, knee, ankle, foot)

G0400 asks whether a resident has a limitation in range of motion (ROM) that interfered with their daily functions or place them at risk for injury. It does **not** ask whether a resident only has a limitation in range of motion. Just having a limitation in ROM doesn't mean that you can code for an impediment.

Tricky parts

Tests for passive range of motion provides no information about a resident's ability to function. You can't use passive tests when coding for this item.

Sometimes residents are unwilling to move their limbs at all. This happens often with residents who have cognitive impairments. In those cases, you should code those extremities as impaired.

Section H: Bladder and bowel

H0200 (urinary toileting program)

H0200: Urinary Toileting Program

Enter Code	**A. Has a trial of a toileting program** (e.g., scheduled toileting, prompted voiding, or bladder training) been attempted on admission/entry or reentry or since urinary incontinence was noted in this facility? 0. **No** → Skip to H0300, Urinary Continence 1. **Yes** → Continue to H0200B, Response 9. **Unable to determine** → Skip to H0200C, Current toileting program or trial
Enter Code	**B. Response** - What was the resident's response to the trial program? 0. **No improvement** 1. **Decreased wetness** 2. **Completely dry** (continent) 9. **Unable to determine** or trial in progress
Enter Code	**C. Current toileting program or trial** - Is a toileting program (e.g., scheduled toileting, prompted voiding, or bladder training) currently being used to manage the resident's urinary continence? 0. **No** 1. **Yes**

Real toileting programs

Common toileting programs are habit training, scheduled voiding, prompted voiding, bladder retraining, and bladder rehabilitation. A toileting program must have:

- a specific approach that is tailored to the resident's unique voiding patterns
- documentation in the care plan
- monitoring
- a written evaluation of the toileting program and resident's responses and progress

Not real toileting programs

Changing pads: Simply tracking continence status, changing pads, and random assistance with toileting are not toileting program interventions.

Initial assessment of toileting skills: Nursing homes will often give newly admitted residents a 72-hour assessment of continence status. This is also not a toileting program. However, it's still important because this assessment will check whether a resident's health status is affecting their continence. Common causes of incontinence are:

- diuretic medications
- urinary tract infections
- vaginitis
- medications that cause lethargy.

A resident who is totally incontinent: If a resident has voiding pattern or is totally incontinent, then they do not qualify for a toileting program. H0200A (urinary toileting program) should be coded 0 (no).

H0100 (appliances)

Lookback period: admission, re-entry, or the date that urinary incontinence was first noticed, whichever is the most recent

H0100. Appliances
↓ Check all that apply
☐ A. **Indwelling catheter** (including suprapubic catheter and nephrostomy tube)
☐ B. **External catheter**
☐ C. **Ostomy** (including urostomy, ileostomy, and colostomy)
☐ D. **Intermittent catheterization**
☐ Z. **None of the above**

During the lookback period, if a resident had an appliance, such as an indwelling catheter or ostomy bag, but then discontinued it, you still have to check it off on H0100. Any appliances used in the last 7 days has to be included.

H0200-C (urinary toileting program or trial)

Lookback period: admission, re-entry, or the date that urinary incontinence was first noticed, whichever is the most recent

H0200. Urinary Toileting Program	
Enter Code	**C. Current toileting program or trial** - Is a toileting program (e.g., scheduled toileting, prompted voiding, or bladder training) currently being used to manage the resident's urinary continence? 0. **No** 1. **Yes**

Code 0 (no, a toileting program is not currently being used)

If a resident is currently in a toileting program, but it was only implemented in 3 or fewer of the last 7 days, then code 0 (no).

If the resident is not on a toileting program, code 0 (no).

Code 1 (yes, a toileting program is currently being used)

If a resident is currently in a toileting program, and it was implemented in 4 or more of the last 7 days, then code 1 (yes).

If a resident participates in a toileting program during the day but prefers not to be awakened to toilet at night, code 1 (yes).

Section I: Active diagnoses

Lookback period: 7 days

Section I is for all of a resident's active diagnoses. Here are some ways to tell whether a diagnosis is an active one or not.

Direct effect on resident's health

An active diagnosis must have a direct relationship to the resident's medical treatments, nursing monitoring, or risk of death. Any clinical documentation of a problem during the 7-day lookback period would be an indication of an active diagnosis. This includes:

- medications
- treatments
- lab and radiology results
- symptoms
- increased monitoring by the nursing staff

Diagnosis by physician

A physician diagnosis is an indication of an active diagnosis. Some state laws allow a nurse practitioner, physician assistant, or clinical nurse specialist to enter in a diagnosis. However, just because a diagnosis is in the diagnosis list doesn't automatically mean that it's an active diagnosis.

Monthly renewal of orders

If a diagnosis is included in a recapped order, then this is an indication that it's an active diagnosis.

....

Inactive diagnoses

Resolved diagnoses that are no longer being treated are inactive diagnoses.

> Providing activity of daily living assistance for functional decline does not count as treating the underlying cause of the functional problems. For example, a resident with a hip fracture wouldn't have an active diagnosis of hip fracture if his only treatment was physical therapy.

I: Active Diagnoses in the Last 7 Days

Active Diagnoses in the last 7 days - Check all that apply
Diagnoses listed in parentheses are provided as examples and should not be considered as all-inclusive lists

Cancer
- ☐ I0100. **Cancer** (with or without metastasis)

Heart/Circulation
- ☐ I0200. **Anemia** (e.g., aplastic, iron deficiency, pernicious, and sickle cell)
- ☐ I0300. **Atrial Fibrillation or Other Dysrhythmias** (e.g., bradycardias and tachycardias)
- ☐ I0400. **Coronary Artery Disease (CAD)** (e.g., angina, myocardial infarction, and atherosclerotic heart disease (ASHD))
- ☐ I0500. **Deep Venous Thrombosis (DVT), Pulmonary Embolus (PE), or Pulmonary Thrombo-Embolism (PTE)**
- ☐ I0600. **Heart Failure** (e.g., congestive heart failure (CHF) and pulmonary edema)
- ☐ I0700. **Hypertension**
- ☐ I0800. **Orthostatic Hypotension**
- ☐ I0900. **Peripheral Vascular Disease (PVD) or Peripheral Arterial Disease (PAD)**

Gastrointestinal
- ☐ I1100. **Cirrhosis**
- ☐ I1200. **Gastroesophageal Reflux Disease (GERD) or Ulcer** (e.g., esophageal, gastric, and peptic ulcers)
- ☐ I1300. **Ulcerative Colitis, Crohn's Disease, or Inflammatory Bowel Disease**

Genitourinary
- ☐ I1400. **Benign Prostatic Hyperplasia (BPH)**
- ☐ I1500. **Renal Insufficiency, Renal Failure, or End-Stage Renal Disease (ESRD)**
- ☐ I1550. **Neurogenic Bladder**
- ☐ I1650. **Obstructive Uropathy**

Infections
- ☐ I1700. **Multidrug-Resistant Organism (MDRO)**
- ☐ I2000. **Pneumonia**
- ☐ I2100. **Septicemia**
- ☐ I2200. **Tuberculosis**
- ☐ I2300. **Urinary Tract Infection (UTI) (LAST 30 DAYS)**
- ☐ I2400. **Viral Hepatitis** (e.g., Hepatitis A, B, C, D, and E)
- ☐ I2500. **Wound Infection** (other than foot)

Metabolic
- ☐ I2900. **Diabetes Mellitus (DM)** (e.g., diabetic retinopathy, nephropathy, and neuropathy)
- ☐ I3100. **Hyponatremia**
- ☐ I3200. **Hyperkalemia**
- ☐ I3300. **Hyperlipidemia** (e.g., hypercholesterolemia)
- ☐ I3400. **Thyroid Disorder** (e.g., hypothyroidism, hyperthyroidism, and Hashimoto's thyroiditis)

Musculoskeletal
- ☐ I3700. **Arthritis** (e.g., degenerative joint disease (DJD), osteoarthritis, and rheumatoid arthritis (RA))
- ☐ I3800. **Osteoporosis**
- ☐ I3900. **Hip Fracture** - any hip fracture that has a relationship to current status, treatments, monitoring (e.g., sub-capital fractures, and fractures of the trochanter and femoral neck)
- ☐ I4000. **Other Fracture**

Neurological
- ☐ I4200. **Alzheimer's Disease**
- ☐ I4300. **Aphasia**
- ☐ I4400. **Cerebral Palsy**
- ☐ I4500. **Cerebrovascular Accident (CVA), Transient Ischemic Attack (TIA), or Stroke**
- ☐ I4800. **Non-Alzheimer's Dementia** (e.g. Lewy body dementia, vascular or multi-infarct dementia; mixed dementia; frontotemporal dementia such as Pick's disease; and dementia related to stroke, Parkinson's or Creutzfeldt-Jakob diseases)

Neurological Diagnoses continued on next page

I: Active Diagnoses in the Last 7 Days (cont.)

Active Diagnoses in the last 7 days - Check all that apply
Diagnoses listed in parentheses are provided as examples and should not be considered as all-inclusive lists

Neurological - Continued
- ☐ I4900. Hemiplegia or Hemiparesis
- ☐ I5000. Paraplegia
- ☐ I5100. Quadriplegia
- ☐ I5200. Multiple Sclerosis (MS)
- ☐ I5250. Huntington's Disease
- ☐ I5300. Parkinson's Disease
- ☐ I5350. Tourette's Syndrome
- ☐ I5400. Seizure Disorder or Epilepsy
- ☐ I5500. Traumatic Brain Injury (TBI)

Nutritional
- ☐ I5600. Malnutrition (protein or calorie) or at risk for malnutrition

Psychiatric/Mood Disorder
- ☐ I5700. Anxiety Disorder
- ☐ I5800. Depression (other than bipolar)
- ☐ I5900. Bipolar Disorder
- ☐ I5950. Psychotic Disorder (other than schizophrenia)
- ☐ I6000. Schizophrenia (e.g., schizoaffective and schizophreniform disorders)
- ☐ I6100. Post Traumatic Stress Disorder (PTSD)

Pulmonary
- ☐ I6200. Asthma, Chronic Obstructive Pulmonary Disease (COPD), or Chronic Lung Disease (e.g., chronic bronchitis and restrictive lung diseases such as asbestosis)
- ☐ I6300. Respiratory Failure

Vision
- ☐ I6500. Cataracts, Glaucoma, or Macular Degeneration

None of Above
- ☐ I7900. None of the above active diagnoses within the last 7 days

Other
I8000. Additional active diagnoses
Enter diagnosis on line and ICD code in boxes. Include the decimal for the code in the appropriate box.

A. _____

B. _____

C. _____

D. _____

E. _____

F. _____

G. _____

H. _____

I. _____

J. _____

I2300 (urinary tract infection)

Lookback period: 30 days

The urinary tract infection (UTI) has its own unique requirements. It uses a 30-day lookback period instead of the standard 7. Additionally, a physician must have entered the diagnosis in the chart within the last 60 days.

Within the last 30 days, a UTI must satisfy these 2 requirements:

1. be diagnosed with an evidence-based criterion such as McGeer, NHSN, or Loeb
2. a physician must have documented the UTI. Some states allow a nurse practitioner, physician assistant, or clinical nurse specialist to also do this.

Infection control

A nursing home's infection prevention and control program (IPCP) has to have routine and systematic surveillance, collection, analysis, and dissemination of data about infections. The criteria for diagnosing UTIs and surveying UTIs in the IPCP should be the same. For example, if the nursing home uses the McGeer criteria to diagnose UTIs bedside, then the IPCP has to also use the McGeer criteria.

Admitted residents who have a diagnosed UTI prior to admission

If a resident comes to the nursing with a UTI already diagnosed, then the nursing home doesn't need to re-evaluate the UTI with their criteria.

If a resident is transferred, but not admitted, to a hospital, then the nursing home has to:

1. use the evidence-based criteria to evaluate whether the resident has a UTI
2. verify that there is a physician-documented UTI diagnosis

Z codes (aftercare codes)

Z codes are used for patients who require continued care for healing, recovery, or long-term care after initial treatment of a disease. A common scenario for Z codes is a resident who needs aftercare after his hospitalization.

When you use a Z code, you should code another diagnosis for a related primary medical condition in I0100-I7900 or entered into I8000.

Tricky parts

Z codes are **not** used in aftercare for traumatic or acute fractures. You should assign a resident with a traumatic fracture a 7th character, such as "D", to indicate a subsequent encounter.

Section J: Health conditions

Section J describes the health conditions that affect a resident's functional status and quality of life.

J0100 (pain management)

Lookback period: 5 days

J0100. Pain Management - Complete for all residents, regardless of current pain level
At any time in the last **5** days, has the resident:

Enter Code ☐   A. **Received scheduled pain medication regimen?**
       0. No
       1. Yes

Enter Code ☐   B. **Received PRN pain medications OR was offered and declined?**
       0. No
       1. Yes

Enter Code ☐   C. **Received non-medication intervention for pain?**
       0. No
       1. Yes

J0100 (pain management) has three items. These are tricky because the labels for the items don't exactly match up with the information that you need to collect.

J0100-A (received scheduled pain medication regimen?)

Enter Code	A. Received scheduled pain medication regimen? 0. No 1. Yes

J0100-A asks whether the resident received their scheduled pain medication.

> If the resident received even one dose of scheduled pain medication was received, code 1 (yes).

> If the resident had orders for scheduled pain medication, but received no scheduled pain medication, code 0 (no).

J0100-B (received PRN pain medications OR was offered and declined?

Enter Code	B. Received PRN pain medications OR was offered and declined? 0. No 1. Yes

J0100-B asks whether the resident received their PRN pain medication or whether they were offered it and declined.

> Even if the resident took no PRN medications during the lookback period, as long as they were offered it and declined, J0100-B is coded 1 (yes).

J0100-C (received non-medication intervention for pain?)

Enter Code	C. Received non-medication intervention for pain? 0. No 1. Yes

J0100-C asks whether the resident received non-medication pain management intervention for pain. If the resident receives a pain medication, then the clinical record must also show an assessment of the pain medication's effectiveness.

Recording all instances of a staff member offering a medication: The facility staff need to consistently document instances of offering medication to residents, even if the resident refuses those medications.

Reason for refusal: When residents refuse to take their medication, it's important to find out why the resident is declining.

Non-pharmacological interventions: When residents have behavioral issues, the nursing home should attempt to use non-pharmacological interventions first. Like medications, staff should document when they offer these interventions and the resident's response.

Common phrases in Section J

Pain medication regimen: A pain medication regimen includes all pharmacological agents that relieve pain or prevent the recurrence of pain. Pain medications can be delivered by oral, transcutaneous, subcutaneous, intramuscular, rectal, intravenous injections, or intraspinal routes.

> The pain medication regimen doesn't include medications that target treatment of underlying conditions, such as chemotherapy or steroids, even if those medications also lead to pain reduction.

Scheduled pain medication regimen: Scheduled drugs have a specific dose and time interval for administration, such as once a day or every 12 hours.

PRN pain medications: Pro re nata medications have a specific dose but are given on an as needed basis. They can have an interval such as "every 6 hours as needed for pain."

J0300 – J0600 (pain assessment interview)

Lookback period: 5 days

This lookback period is shorter than the others because the pain interview requires the resident to recall specific information. CMS says that you should conduct this interview close to the end of the 5-day lookback period, preferably on the ARD or the day before the ARD.

Questions: The pain assessment interview has questions about:

- the presence (J0300)
- frequency of pain (J0400)
- effect of the pain on the resident's function (J0500)
- intensity of pain (J0600) of pain

Pain Assessment Interview	
J0300. Pain Presence	
Enter Code	Ask resident: "***Have you had pain or hurting at any time*** in the last 5 days?" 0. **No** → Skip to J1100, Shortness of Breath 1. **Yes** → Continue to J0400, Pain Frequency 9. **Unable to answer** → Skip to J0800, Indicators of Pain or Possible Pain
J0400. Pain Frequency	
Enter Code	Ask resident: "***How much of the time have you experienced pain or hurting*** over the last 5 days?" 1. **Almost constantly** 2. **Frequently** 3. **Occasionally** 4. **Rarely** 9. **Unable to answer**
J0500. Pain Effect on Function	
Enter Code	**A.** Ask resident: "*Over the past 5 days,* **has pain made it hard for you to sleep at night?**" 0. **No** 1. **Yes** 9. **Unable to answer**
Enter Code	**B.** Ask resident: "*Over the past 5 days,* **have you limited your day-to-day activities because of pain?**" 0. **No** 1. **Yes** 9. **Unable to answer**
J0600. Pain Intensity - Administer **ONLY ONE** of the following pain intensity questions (A or B)	
Enter Rating	**A. Numeric Rating Scale (00-10)** Ask resident: "*Please rate your worst pain over the last 5 days on a zero to ten scale, with zero being no pain and ten as the worst pain you can imagine.*" (Show resident 00-10 pain scale) **Enter two-digit response. Enter 99 if unable to answer.**
Enter Code	**B. Verbal Descriptor Scale** Ask resident: "*Please rate the intensity of your worst pain over the last 5 days.*" (Show resident verbal scale) 1. **Mild** 2. **Moderate** 3. **Severe** 4. **Very severe, horrible** 9. **Unable to answer**

Conducting pain interview with all residents

Nursing home staff should attempt to conduct the pain interview with all residents.

If the resident isn't able to answer J0300 (pain presence), stop the interview, skip the remaining questions, and do the staff assessment for pain instead.

When the interview does go forward but at some point the resident chooses not to answer, is unable to answer a question, does not respond, or gives a nonsensical response to the question, select the code 9 and go to the next question.

B0700 (makes self understood)

B0700: Makes Self Understood

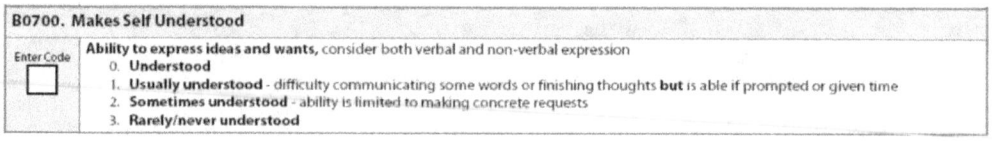

Although J0300 (the pain interview) isn't related to B0700 (makes self understood), surveyors may look at discrepancies between the two.

Definition of pain

Pain is defined however the resident defines it. Residents may not find the term "pain" useful, so the interviewer can also use words like hurting, aching, soreness, burning, discomfort, and so on. The information from the resident's response is used in J0300, J0400, J0500, and J0600.

Other information sources

The pain interview is only one source of information for the pain assessment. Staff observations and clinical assessment are also taken into consideration when making care plans.

J1550: Problem Conditions

	J1550. Problem Conditions	
	↓ Check all that apply	
☐	A.	Fever
☐	B.	Vomiting
☐	C.	Dehydrated
☐	D.	Internal bleeding
☐	Z.	None of the above

J1550-A (fever)

A fever is a temperature 2.4°F higher than the resident's baseline temperature.

If the nursing home hasn't taken a baseline temperature, then a fever is 100.4°F.

J1550-C (dehydrated)

Dehydration must fulfill at least two of the following:

- The resident usually takes in less than the recommended 1,500 ml of fluids per day
- Resident has one or more clinical signs of dehydration
- Resident's fluid loss exceeds the amount of fluids he takes in. Common causes of this include vomiting, fever, diarrhea

J1700 (fall history on admission/entry or reentry)

A **fall** is an unintentional change in position that ends with the resident on the ground, floor, or onto the next lower surface, such as a bed, chair, or bedside mat.

Clinical record: Nursing facilities need to have a full record of all a resident's falls. Staff members should be trained to recognize falls and nurses should interview various staff members on all shifts to find out if anyone fell.

> **Time**: Falls can be witnessed live or the resident can be later found on the floor or ground.
>
> **Location**: Falls don't have to occur only in the nursing home. They can also occur at home, outside in the community, or in a hospital. Nursing homes should get clinical records from the hospital and see if the resident fell while in their acute stay.
>
> **Intercepted falls**: If someone catches a resident before they fall, and the resident would not have caught themselves without their help, then that still counts as a fall.

Falls during therapy: Nursing homes often will provide therapeutic intervention that challenge a resident's balance. Falls that happen in these circumstances don't count as falls.

Falls from altercations: Falls that occur because of an overwhelming external force, such a resident pushing another resident, don't count as falls.

J1700. Fall History on Admission/Entry or Reentry		
Complete only if A0310A = 01 or A0310E = 1		
Enter Code	**A.**	Did the resident have a fall any time in the **last month** prior to admission/entry or reentry? 0. **No** 1. **Yes** 9. **Unable to determine**
Enter Code	**B.**	Did the resident have a fall any time in the **last 2-6 months** prior to admission/entry or reentry? 0. **No** 1. **Yes** 9. **Unable to determine**
Enter Code	**C.**	Did the resident have any **fracture related to a fall in the 6 months** prior to admission/entry or reentry? 0. **No** 1. **Yes** 9. **Unable to determine**

J1800 (falls since admission)

Section J1800 counts the number of falls since a resident's admission, entry, reentry, prior OBRA assessment, or scheduled PPS, whichever is more recent.

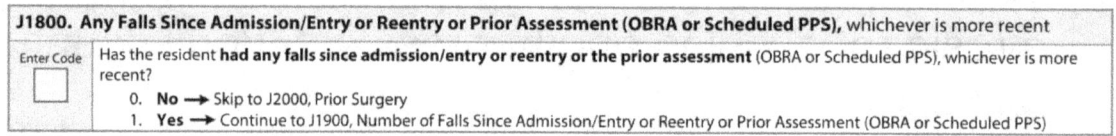

Assessments completed but not submitted: If a resident had a prospective payment system (PPS) assessment done for an insurance other than Medicare A, but this assessment wasn't submitted, then it can't be used for J1800.

> **PPS assessments**: The schedule for Medicare-required PPS assessments is at day 5, 14, 30, 60, and 90. There are also additional unscheduled assessments for certain circumstances.

J1900-C (number of falls with major injury)

Lookback period: the most recent admission, entry, re-entry, or prior assessment

Section J1900-C counts the number of falls that result in a major injury. Major injuries include bone fractures, joint dislocations, or closed head injuries with altered consciousness or subdural hematoma. Subdural hematomas are major injuries, whether or not there was altered consciousness.

> If a resident has a closed head injury, but it isn't a subdural hematoma, then it must have resulted in altered consciousness to be included as a major injury.

Tricky parts

In addition to the usual clinical records, like home incident reports, fall logs, and the medical record, the resident and their family are a good source of information about falls and injuries. Information from them is valid, even if it wasn't initially documented in the medical record.

Section K: Swallowing and nutritional status

Lookback period: 30 and 180 days

Since October 2019, A0510-C (mechanically altered diet) and K0510-D (therapeutic diet) are no longer included in for K0510.

K0300: Weight Loss

K0300. Weight Loss	
Enter Code	Loss of 5% or more in the last month or loss of 10% or more in last 6 months 0. **No** or unknown 1. **Yes, on** physician-prescribed weight-loss regimen 2. **Yes, not on** physician-prescribed weight-loss regimen

Section K covers swallowing disorders, height and weight, weight loss, and nutritional approaches. **Weight loss** is defined as a weight loss of 5% or more in the past 30 days or 10% or more in the last 180 days.

No previous weight: The nursing staff usually get weight information from the clinical record. If a resident's last recorded weight was taken over 30 days before or it isn't available, then the staff should weight the resident again before the ARD.

K0510 (nutritional approaches)

Lookback period: 7 days

K0510: Nutritional Approaches

K0510. Nutritional Approaches — Check all of the following nutritional approaches that were performed during the last **7 days**	1. While NOT a Resident	2. While a Resident
1. While NOT a Resident — Performed *while NOT a resident* of this facility and within the *last 7 days*. Only check column 1 if resident entered (admission or reentry) IN THE LAST 7 DAYS. If resident last entered 7 or more days ago, leave column 1 blank. **2. While a Resident** — Performed *while a resident* of this facility and within the *last 7 days*	↓ Check all that apply ↓	
A. Parenteral/IV feeding	☐	☐
B. Feeding tube - nasogastric or abdominal (PEG)	☐	☐
C. Mechanically altered diet - require change in texture of food or liquids (e.g., pureed food, thickened liquids)	▓	☐
D. Therapeutic diet (e.g., low salt, diabetic, low cholesterol)	▓	☐
Z. None of the above	☐	☐

Section K510 is for a resident's nutrition and hydration items that were administered for nutrition and hydration. This section is also separated into the nutrition and hydration items that the patient received while they were a resident at the nursing home and while they weren't.

Tricky parts

The medical record has to document why a resident needs a particular nutritional approach.

- The nursing home attempted standard nutrition and hydration approaches
- Standard approaches were found to be insufficient for the resident's needs

K0510-A (parenteral/IV feeding)

Some IV fluids can be coded into K510-A (parenteral/IV feeding) if the medical record shows that the resident has a clinical nutrition or hydration need and requires additional fluid intake. The following fluids can be included:

- IV fluids or hyperalimentation, including total parenteral nutrition (TPN), administered continuously or intermittently
- IV fluids running at KVO (keep vein open)
- IV fluids contained in IV piggybacks
- Hypodermoclysis and subcutaneous ports in hydration therapy
- IV fluids given specifically for prevention of dehydration

The following items do **not** belong in K0510-A:

- IV medications, these belong in O0100-H (IV medications)
- IV fluids used to reconstitute or dilute medications for IV administration
- IV fluids administered as a routine part of an operative or diagnostic procedure or recovery room stay
- IV fluids administered solely as flushes
- Parenteral/IV fluids administered in conjunction with chemotherapy or dialysis

Enteral feeding formulas

You can code enteral formulas for tube feedings under K0510-D (therapeutic diet) if the formula was altered to manage a problematic health condition, such as diabetes.

You should **not** code enteral feeding formulas as a mechanically altered diet.

K0710 (percent intake by artificial route)

Lookback period: 7 days

K0710: Percent Intake by Artificial Route

Complete K0710 only if Column 1 and/or Column 2 are checked for K0510A and/or K0510B.

K0710. Percent Intake by Artificial Route - Complete K0710 only if Column 1 and/or Column 2 are checked for K0510A and/or K0510B.	2. While a Resident	3. During Entire 7 Days
2. While a Resident — Performed *while a resident* of this facility and within the *last 7 days* **3. During Entire 7 Days** — Performed during the entire *last 7 days*	↓ Enter Codes ↓	
A. Proportion of total calories the resident received through parenteral or tube feeding 1. 25% or less 2. 26-50% 3. 51% or more	☐	☐
B. Average fluid intake per day by IV or tube feeding 1. 500 cc/day or less 2. 501 cc/day or more	☐	☐

Item K0710 is the proportion of total calories the resident received through either parenteral or tube feeding, as well as the average fluid intake per day by either IV or tube feeding.

This section is divided into two columns. One column is for whether the patient received parenteral or tube feeding while he was a resident, and the other column is for whether the patient received parenteral or tube feeding during the entire 7 days.

Section M: Skin conditions

Lookback period: 7 days

M0210. Unhealed Pressure Ulcers/Injuries
Enter Code   Does this resident have one or more unhealed pressure ulcers/injuries?
0. **No** → Skip to M1030, Number of Venous and Arterial Ulcers
1. **Yes** → Continue to M0300, Current Number of Unhealed Pressure Ulcers/Injuries at Each Stage

M0210 (unhealed pressure injuries)

Section M02010 shows whether or not a resident had one or more unhealed pressure injuries. A **pressure injury** is a localized injury to the skin or its underlying tissue, as a result of pressure or sheer. Pressure injuries must have pressure as the primary cause. Injuries with different etiologies should be coded in other sections.

> **Healed ulcers**: If a resident had a pressure wound, but it healed during the look-back period, then it doesn't need to be included in this section.

M0300 (current number of unhealed pressure injuries at each stage)

	M0300. Current Number of Unhealed Pressure Ulcers/Injuries at Each Stage
Enter Number ☐	**A. Stage 1:** Intact skin with non-blanchable redness of a localized area usually over a bony prominence. Darkly pigmented skin may not have a visible blanching; in dark skin tones only it may appear with persistent blue or purple hues **1. Number of Stage 1 pressure injuries**
Enter Number ☐	**B. Stage 2:** Partial thickness loss of dermis presenting as a shallow open ulcer with a red or pink wound bed, without slough. May also present as an intact or open/ruptured blister **1. Number of Stage 2 pressure ulcers** - If 0 → Skip to M0300C, Stage 3
Enter Number ☐	**2. Number of these Stage 2 pressure ulcers that were present upon admission/entry or reentry** - enter how many were noted at the time of admission/entry or reentry
Enter Number ☐	**C. Stage 3:** Full thickness tissue loss. Subcutaneous fat may be visible but bone, tendon or muscle is not exposed. Slough may be present but does not obscure the depth of tissue loss. May include undermining and tunneling **1. Number of Stage 3 pressure ulcers** - If 0 → Skip to M0300D, Stage 4
Enter Number ☐	**2. Number of these Stage 3 pressure ulcers that were present upon admission/entry or reentry** - enter how many were noted at the time of admission/entry or reentry
Enter Number ☐	**D. Stage 4:** Full thickness tissue loss with exposed bone, tendon or muscle. Slough or eschar may be present on some parts of the wound bed. Often includes undermining and tunneling **1. Number of Stage 4 pressure ulcers** - If 0 → Skip to M0300E, Unstageable - Non-removable dressing/device
Enter Number ☐	**2. Number of these Stage 4 pressure ulcers that were present upon admission/entry or reentry** - enter how many were noted at the time of admission/entry or reentry
Enter Number ☐	**E. Unstageable - Non-removable dressing/device:** Known but not stageable due to non-removable dressing/device **1. Number of unstageable pressure ulcers/injuries due to non-removable dressing/device** - If 0 → Skip to M0300F, Unstageable - Slough and/or eschar
Enter Number ☐	**2. Number of these unstageable pressure ulcers/injuries that were present upon admission/entry or reentry** - enter how many were noted at the time of admission/entry or reentry
Enter Number ☐	**F. Unstageable - Slough and/or eschar:** Known but not stageable due to coverage of wound bed by slough and/or eschar **1. Number of unstageable pressure ulcers due to coverage of wound bed by slough and/or eschar** - If 0 → Skip to M0300G, Unstageable - Deep tissue injury
Enter Number ☐	**2. Number of these unstageable pressure ulcers that were present upon admission/entry or reentry** - enter how many were noted at the time of admission/entry or reentry
Enter Number ☐	**G. Unstageable - Deep tissue injury:** **1. Number of unstageable pressure injuries presenting as deep tissue injury** - If 0 → Skip to M1030, Number of Venous and Arterial Ulcers
Enter Number ☐	**2. Number of these unstageable pressure injuries that were present upon admission/entry or reentry** - enter how many were noted at the time of admission/entry or reentry

M0300-A (stage 1 pressure injuries)

M0300A: Number of Stage 1 Pressure Injuries

M0300. Current Number of Unhealed Pressure Ulcers/Injuries at Each Stage
A. Stage 1: Intact skin with non-blanchable redness of a localized area usually over a bony prominence. Darkly pigmented skin may not have a visible blanching; in dark skin tones only it may appear with persistent blue or purple hues
Enter Number ☐   1. Number of Stage 1 pressure injuries

A stage 1 pressure injury is a superficial reddening of the skin.

It's easy to confuse a **pressure injury** and a **deep tissue injury**. Both of them use the temperature (warmth and coolness) and tissue consistency (firm and boggy) descriptors. I'm going to be honest: I don't know how to tell the difference between the two either. So, hopefully you already know how to do that.

> **Darker skin**: It can be difficult to assess pressure injuries on residents with darker skin tones. Color changes such as persistent red, blue, or purple hues indicate a pressure injury. A change in temperature is also a sign of a pressure injury.

M0300-B (stage 2 pressure injuries)

M0300B: Stage 2 Pressure Ulcers

B. Stage 2: Partial thickness loss of dermis presenting as a shallow open ulcer with a red or pink wound bed, without slough. May also present as an intact or open/ruptured blister

Enter Number ☐ 1. **Number of Stage 2 pressure ulcers** - If 0 → Skip to M0300C, Stage 3

Enter Number ☐ 2. **Number of these Stage 2 pressure ulcers that were present upon admission/entry or reentry** - enter how many were noted at the time of admission/entry or reentry

A stage 2 pressure injury is a partial thickness loss of dermis. This injury can present as a shallow, open ulcer with a red-pink wound bed, without slough or bruising, or as an intact blister. Stage 2 pressure injuries do not have granulation tissue, slough, or eschar.

Healing: Most stage 2 pressure injuries heal in a reasonable time frame, such as 60 days. If the pressure injury doesn't heal within 14 days, the staff should re-assess the resident's overall condition.

M0300-C (stage 3 pressure injuries)

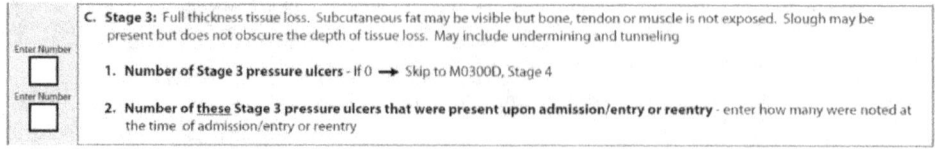

A stage 3 pressure ulcer is full thickness skin loss that has damage or necrosis of subcutaneous tissue down to the underlying fascia. It looks like a deep crater with or without undermining of adjacent tissue. Bones, tendons, and muscle will not be visible or directly palpable in a stage 3 pressure injury.

M0300-D (stage 4 pressure injuries)

M0300D: Stage 4 Pressure Ulcers

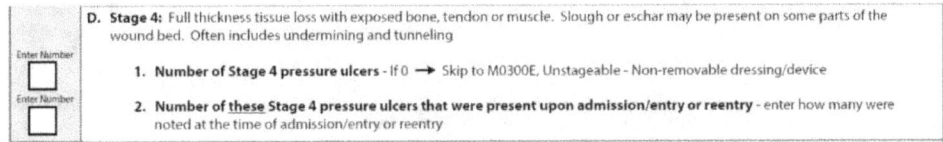

A stage 4 pressure ulcer is full thickness skin loss with extensive destruction, tissue necrosis, or damage to muscle, bone, or supporting structures. These ulcers may also have undermining and sinus tracts. Pressure injuries that have exposed cartilage should be classified as stage 4.

Section N: Medications

Lookback period: 7 days

N0410. Medications Received
Indicate the number of DAYS the resident received the following medications by pharmacological classification, not how it is used, during the last 7 days or since admission/entry or reentry if less than 7 days. Enter "0" if medication was not received by the resident during the last 7 days
Enter Days ☐ A. Antipsychotic
Enter Days ☐ B. Antianxiety
Enter Days ☐ C. Antidepressant
Enter Days ☐ D. Hypnotic
Enter Days ☐ E. Anticoagulant (e.g., warfarin, heparin, or low-molecular weight heparin)
Enter Days ☐ F. Antibiotic
Enter Days ☐ G. Diuretic
Enter Days ☐ H. Opioid

N0410 (medications received)

Section N0410 shows the number of days that a resident received medications. The subsections in N0410 are organized by **pharmacological classification**, not by how the resident uses it.

> **Oxazepam**: For example, oxazepam is an anti-anxiety medication, but some people use it to sleep better. However, it has to be classified by his pharmacological class, not its use. Therefore, it is an anti-anxiety medication, not a hypnotic.

Section N0410 also includes medications received by all routes and settings. Here are some of the most common routes and settings.

Routes: oral (PO), intramuscular (IM), intravenous (IV)

Settings: nursing facility, hospital emergency room

Section O: Special treatments, procedures, and programs

O0100-M (isolation or quarantine for active infectious disease)

Section O0100-M is important because it's one of the few items that can classify a resident into a higher-paying case-mix group for Medicare Part A. It records the most labor-intensive levels of isolation. However, the definitions for section O0100-M change regularly, so it's tricky to code right.

If a nursing facility wants to code a resident as requiring **single room isolation**, it has to show that it's for the protection of both the resident and other people. CMS determines whether a resident needs isolation on a case-by-case basis, but generally, the resident must fulfill these requirements to be considered:

- **Resident is very sick**: The resident has an active infection with highly transmissible or epidemiologically significant pathogens.

- **Pathogen is very contagious**: The pathogen can be acquired by physical contact, airborne transmission, or droplet transmission.
- **Extra precautions**: The staff have to take above standard precautions, such as contact precautions, droplet precautions, or airborne precautions.
- **Resident can't have a roommate**: The resident has to be in a room alone. It doesn't matter whether the roommate has a similar infection and also requires isolation.
- **Resident can't leave his room**: The resident has to stay in his room and all services have to be brought to him. This includes dining, activities, and rehabilitation.

O0100: Special Treatments, Procedures, and Programs

Facilities may code treatments, programs and procedures that the resident performed themselves independently or after set-up by facility staff. Do not code services that were provided solely in conjunction with a surgical procedure or diagnostic procedure, such as IV medications or ventilators. Surgical procedures include routine pre- and post-operative procedures.

O0100. Special Treatments, Procedures, and Programs		
Check all of the following treatments, procedures, and programs that were performed during the last **14 days**		
1. While NOT a Resident Performed *while NOT a resident* of this facility and within the *last 14 days*. Only check column 1 if resident entered (admission or reentry) IN THE LAST 14 DAYS. If resident last entered 14 or more days ago, leave column 1 blank **2. While a Resident** Performed *while a resident* of this facility and within the *last 14 days*	**1.** While NOT a Resident	**2.** While a Resident
	↓ Check all that apply ↓	
Cancer Treatments		
A. **Chemotherapy**	☐	☐
B. **Radiation**	☐	☐
Respiratory Treatments		
C. **Oxygen therapy**	☐	☐
D. **Suctioning**	☐	☐
E. **Tracheostomy care**	☐	☐
F. **Invasive Mechanical Ventilator** (ventilator or respirator)	☐	☐
G. **Non-Invasive Mechanical Ventilator** (BiPAP/CPAP)	☐	☐
Other		
H. **IV medications**	☐	☐
I. **Transfusions**	☐	☐
J. **Dialysis**	☐	☐
K. **Hospice care**	☐	☐
M. **Isolation or quarantine for active infectious disease** (does not include standard body/fluid precautions)	☐	☐
None of the Above		
Z. **None of the above**	☐	☐

Exceptions to single room isolation

Isolation criteria don't apply to:

- urinary tract infections
- encapsulated pneumonia
- wound infections

Emergency treatments

If a resident meets the criteria for single room isolation but has to leave the facility for critical medical treatment that can't be postponed, this does not disqualify the resident from O0100-M. Both the transport vehicle and the receiving facility staff have to take appropriate precautions.

Reverse isolation

O0100-M is not for reverse isolation. Reverse isolation is when the resident doesn't have an active infection, but the nursing home wants to protect him from pathogens that others may transmit.

O0300 (pneumococcal vaccine)

Item O0300 records whether a resident's pneumococcal vaccine is up to date.

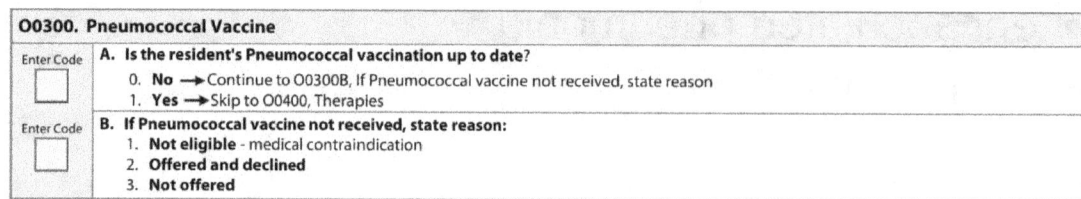

There are two types of pneumococcal vaccines:

- pneumococcal conjugate vaccine (PCV13 or Prevnar13)
- pneumococcal polysaccharide vaccine (PPSV23 or Pneumovax23)

Adults 19 to 64 with cerebrospinal fluid leaks or cochlear implants: These people should get 1 dose of PCV13 and then wait at least 8 weeks for a PPSV23 booster shot.

Adults 19 to 64 with immunodeficiencies: These people should get 1 dose of PCV13, then wait at least 8 weeks for 1 PPSV23 booster shot, and then wait 5 years for a second PPSV23 booster shot.

Anyone who smokes: These people should get 1 dose of PPSV23.

Anyone who has heart disease, alcoholism, liver disease, lung disease, or diabetes: These people should get 1 dose of PPSV23.

Adults 65 and older with no immunodeficiencies: For people aged 65 and older and who have no immunodeficiencies, the recommended first dose is the PPSV23 vaccine. They should then wait 5 years for a PPSV23 booster shot.

For adults over 65 who don't have immunodeficiencies and also want to receive both the PCV13 and the PPSV23, they should get the PCV13 first and then wait at least 1 year for the PPSV23 booster shot.

Older adults with immunodeficiencies: For people age 65 and older and who have immunodeficiencies, the recommended first dose is the PCV13 vaccine. They should then wait 8 weeks for a PPSV23 booster shot.

Nursing home residents may benefit more from the PCV13 vaccine.

Booster shots: If a resident received their first dose of the pneumococcal vaccine, but it isn't yet time for their booster shot, it still counts as an up-to-date pneumococcal vaccine.

For example, if a 70-year-old resident with no immunodeficiencies got the PCV13 vaccine 6 months prior to admission, this would be coded as O0300 = 1 (yes). They still have 4.5 years until their next scheduled vaccine.

O0400 (therapies)

Section O0400 is for speech, occupational, and physical therapy. Only skilled therapy can go in this section.

O0400: Therapies

O0400. Therapies	
A. Speech-Language Pathology and Audiology Services	
Enter Number of Minutes	1. **Individual minutes** - record the total number of minutes this therapy was administered to the resident **individually** in the last 7 days
Enter Number of Minutes	2. **Concurrent minutes** - record the total number of minutes this therapy was administered to the resident **concurrently with one other resident** in the last 7 days
Enter Number of Minutes	3. **Group minutes** - record the total number of minutes this therapy was administered to the resident as **part of a group of residents** in the last 7 days
	If the sum of individual, concurrent, and group minutes is zero, → skip to O0400A5, Therapy start date
Enter Number of Minutes	3A. **Co-treatment minutes** - record the total number of minutes this therapy was administered to the resident in **co-treatment sessions** in the last 7 days
Enter Number of Days	4. **Days** - record the **number of days** this therapy was administered for **at least 15 minutes** a day in the last 7 days
5. **Therapy start date** - record the date the most recent therapy regimen (since the most recent entry) started Month - Day - Year	6. **Therapy end date** - record the date the most recent therapy regimen (since the most recent entry) ended - enter dashes if therapy is ongoing Month - Day - Year
B. Occupational Therapy	
Enter Number of Minutes	1. **Individual minutes** - record the total number of minutes this therapy was administered to the resident **individually** in the last 7 days
Enter Number of Minutes	2. **Concurrent minutes** - record the total number of minutes this therapy was administered to the resident **concurrently with one other resident** in the last 7 days
Enter Number of Minutes	3. **Group minutes** - record the total number of minutes this therapy was administered to the resident as **part of a group of residents** in the last 7 days
	If the sum of individual, concurrent, and group minutes is zero, → skip to O0400B5, Therapy start date
Enter Number of Minutes	3A. **Co-treatment minutes** - record the total number of minutes this therapy was administered to the resident in **co-treatment sessions** in the last 7 days
Enter Number of Days	4. **Days** - record the **number of days** this therapy was administered for **at least 15 minutes** a day in the last 7 days
5. **Therapy start date** - record the date the most recent therapy regimen (since the most recent entry) started Month - Day - Year	6. **Therapy end date** - record the date the most recent therapy regimen (since the most recent entry) ended - enter dashes if therapy is ongoing Month - Day - Year
O0400 continued on next page	

O0400: Therapies (cont.)

O0400. Therapies - Continued

C. Physical Therapy

Enter Number of Minutes
1. **Individual minutes** - record the total number of minutes this therapy was administered to the resident **individually** in the last 7 days

Enter Number of Minutes
2. **Concurrent minutes** - record the total number of minutes this therapy was administered to the resident **concurrently with one other resident** in the last 7 days

Enter Number of Minutes
3. **Group minutes** - record the total number of minutes this therapy was administered to the resident as **part of a group of residents** in the last 7 days

If the sum of individual, concurrent, and group minutes is zero, → skip to O0400C5, Therapy start date

Enter Number of Minutes
3A. **Co-treatment minutes** - record the total number of minutes this therapy was administered to the resident in **co-treatment sessions** in the last 7 days

Enter Number of Days
4. **Days** - record the **number of days** this therapy was administered for **at least 15 minutes** a day in the last 7 days

5. **Therapy start date** - record the date the most recent therapy regimen (since the most recent entry) started

6. **Therapy end date** - record the date the most recent therapy regimen (since the most recent entry) ended - enter dashes if therapy is ongoing

[ ][ ] - [ ][ ] - [ ][ ][ ][ ]   [ ][ ] - [ ][ ] - [ ][ ][ ][ ]
Month Day   Year   Month Day   Year

D. Respiratory Therapy

Enter Number of Minutes
1. **Total minutes** - record the total number of minutes this therapy was administered to the resident in the last 7 days
If zero, → skip to O0400E, Psychological Therapy

Enter Number of Days
2. **Days** - record the **number of days** this therapy was administered for **at least 15 minutes** a day in the last 7 days

E. Psychological Therapy (by any licensed mental health professional)

Enter Number of Minutes
1. **Total minutes** - record the total number of minutes this therapy was administered to the resident in the last 7 days
If zero, → skip to O0400F, Recreational Therapy

Enter Number of Days
2. **Days** - record the **number of days** this therapy was administered for **at least 15 minutes** a day in the last 7 days

F. Recreational Therapy (includes recreational and music therapy)

Enter Number of Minutes
1. **Total minutes** - record the total number of minutes this therapy was administered to the resident in the last 7 days
If zero, → skip to O0420, Distinct Calendar Days of Therapy

Enter Number of Days
2. **Days** - record the **number of days** this therapy was administered for **at least 15 minutes** a day in the last 7 days

Skilled therapy: Skilled therapy is therapy that requires the skills of a therapist. If the therapy services can be provided by non-skilled personnel, then it isn't skilled therapy. The resident's potential for recovery doesn't matter.

Therapy start date:

Therapy can start anytime between the date at A1600 and the current day.

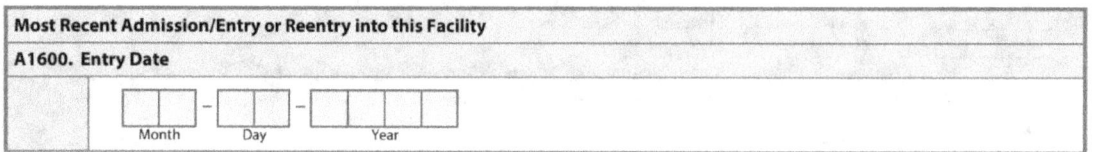

The therapy start date is the date that a resident's therapy regimen started. If the resident had more than one therapy regimen since A1600, then the therapy start date is the start date of the most recent therapy regimen.

Therapy end date: The therapy end date is the last date that the resident received skilled therapy treatment.

The end date means the date that the most recent therapy regimen ended, so if the resident's treatment is still ongoing, then code dashes for therapy end date.

Ongoing therapy: Therapy is considered ongoing if the resident is still in the middle of his therapy regimen.

Here are some more common scenarios for ongoing therapy:

- The resident was discharged, and his therapy was planned to continue if the resident had remained in the facility
- The resident's SNF benefit exhausted, but the nursing home still provided his therapy
- The resident's payer source changed, and the nursing home continued to provide him with therapy

Section P: Restraints and alarms

Physical restraints restrict a resident's freedom of movement or normal access to their body. It can be manual method or a physical device, material, or equipment. The physical restraint can be attached to or adjacent to the resident's body.

Section P	Restraints and Alarms
P0100. Physical Restraints	
Physical restraints are any manual method or physical or mechanical device, material or equipment attached or adjacent to the resident's body that the individual cannot remove easily which restricts freedom of movement or normal access to one's body	

	↓ Enter Codes in Boxes
	Used in Bed
Coding:	A. Bed rail
0. Not used	B. Trunk restraint
1. Used less than daily	C. Limb restraint
2. Used daily	D. Other
	Used in Chair or Out of Bed
	E. Trunk restraint
	F. Limb restraint
	G. Chair prevents rising
	H. Other

P0200. Alarms		
An alarm is any physical or electronic device that monitors resident movement and alerts the staff when movement is detected		
	↓ Enter Codes in Boxes	
Coding: 0. Not used 1. Used less than daily 2. Used daily	☐	A. Bed alarm
	☐	B. Chair alarm
	☐	C. Floor mat alarm
	☐	D. Motion sensor alarm
	☐	E. Wander/elopement alarm
	☐	F. Other alarm

People often think of restraints as handcuffs or ropes, but ordinary objects can also be considered restraints. On the other hand, what is considered a restraint for one resident may not be considered a restraint for another resident. It's important to make an interdisciplinary assessment of a resident's functional and psychological strengths and limitations before deeming something a restraint or not.

Here are two cases where a chair was and wasn't a restraint:

- A resident requires a staff member to transfer and bear weight. He likes to sit in a reclining, wheeled lounge chair, but he is incapable of self-transfer when the chair is in the recumbent position. While in the chair, the resident attempts to unsafely transfer by himself by putting his seat on the side of the chair, scooting to the edge of the chair, and holding himself up with his hands. In this case, the

chair is a restraint because it is preventing the resident from standing up.
- A resident requires two staff members and a Hoyer lift to transfer. She has no voluntary movement at all. She sits in the same reclining chair as the resident above but makes no movement that indicates she wants to get up. In this case, the chair would not be considered a restraint because it isn't preventing her from standing up.

Here are two cases where a "lap buddy" was and wasn't a restraint:

- A resident at high risk of falls often impulsively rises from her wheelchair. Her wheelchair has a lap buddy, which is a foam device that goes between the arm rests and her from getting up. The resident occasionally tries to remove the device by wiggling the device. After a few minutes, she succeeds and pulls it off the side of the wheelchair. This device would be considered a restraint.
- A resident at high risk of falls often impulsively rises from his wheelchair. He also has a lap buddy. However, he is able to remove the device easily and has a regular schedule for when he has a lap buddy. When state asks him what it's for, he tells them that it's to keep him from falling out of his wheelchair. This device would not be considered a restraint.

Section V: Care area assessment (CAA) summary

Some responses to MDS items will automatically signal a problem area, which then requires additional assessment. This is called a **triggered care area**. The interdisciplinary team and the resident then decided whether to develop a care plan for the triggered care areas.

Nursing homes have to document the **care area assessments** (**CAAs**) that were triggered and the care plans that resulted from them. State surveyors think this is very important.

Section V also documents some prior assessment items that relate to care area assessments.

Care area assessments (CAAs)

There are 20 care area assessments in the resident assessment instrument, version 3.0.

1. Delirium
2. Cognitive loss, dementia
3. Visual function
4. Communication
5. Activity of daily living (ADL) functional and rehabilitation potential
6. Urinary incontinence and indwelling catheter
7. Psychosocial well-being
8. Mood state
9. Behavioral symptoms
10. Activities
11. Falls
12. Nutritional status
13. Feeding tubes
14. Dehydration, fluid maintenance
15. Dental care
16. Pressure ulcer
17. Psychotropic medication use
18. Physical restraints
19. Pain
20. Return to community referral

Care area trigger (CAT) logic tables

Each separate CAA has certain criteria before it is triggered. The specific criteria are called the **care area trigger (CAT) logic tables**. I won't go over all of them because some of them are quite long, but I will go over the communication logic table.

B0200. Hearing

Enter Code

Ability to hear (with hearing aid or hearing appliances if normally used)
0. **Adequate** - no difficulty in normal conversation, social interaction, listening to TV
1. **Minimal difficulty** - difficulty in some environments (e.g., when person speaks softly or setting is noisy)
2. **Moderate difficulty** - speaker has to increase volume and speak distinctly
3. **Highly impaired** - absence of useful hearing

B0700. Makes Self Understood

Enter Code

Ability to express ideas and wants, consider both verbal and non-verbal expression
0. **Understood**
1. **Usually understood** - difficulty communicating some words or finishing thoughts **but** is able if prompted or given time
2. **Sometimes understood** - ability is limited to making concrete requests
3. **Rarely/never understood**

B0800. Ability To Understand Others

Enter Code

Understanding verbal content, however able (with hearing aid or device if used)
0. **Understands** - clear comprehension
1. **Usually understands** - misses some part/intent of message **but** comprehends most conversation
2. **Sometimes understands** - responds adequately to simple, direct communication only
3. **Rarely/never understands**

Care area trigger logic table		
Clinical significance	Triggering conditions	Name of item
Hearing problems	B0200 ≥ 1 and B0200 ≥ 3	Hearing
Impaired ability to make self understood	B0700 ≥ 1 and B0700 ≤ 3	Makes self understood
Impaired ability to understand others	B0800 ≥1 and B0800 ≤3	Ability to understand others

Section V — Care Area Assessment (CAA) Summary

V0200. CAAs and Care Planning

1. Check column A if Care Area is triggered.
2. For each triggered Care Area, indicate whether a new care plan, care plan revision, or continuation of current care plan is necessary to address the problem(s) identified in your assessment of the care area. The Care Planning Decision column must be completed within 7 days of completing the RAI (MDS and CAA(s)). Check column B if the triggered care area is addressed in the care plan.
3. Indicate in the Location and Date of CAA Documentation column where information related to the CAA can be found. CAA documentation should include information on the complicating factors, risks, and any referrals for this resident for this care area.

A. CAA Results

Care Area	A. Care Area Triggered	B. Care Planning Decision	Location and Date of CAA documentation
	↓ Check all that apply ↓		
01. Delirium	☐	☐	
02. Cognitive Loss/Dementia	☐	☐	
03. Visual Function	☐	☐	
04. Communication	☐	☐	
05. ADL Functional/Rehabilitation Potential	☐	☐	
06. Urinary Incontinence and Indwelling Catheter	☐	☐	
07. Psychosocial Well-Being	☐	☐	
08. Mood State	☐	☐	
09. Behavioral Symptoms	☐	☐	
10. Activities	☐	☐	
11. Falls	☐	☐	
12. Nutritional Status	☐	☐	
13. Feeding Tube	☐	☐	
14. Dehydration/Fluid Maintenance	☐	☐	
15. Dental Care	☐	☐	
16. Pressure Ulcer	☐	☐	
17. Psychotropic Drug Use	☐	☐	
18. Physical Restraints	☐	☐	
19. Pain	☐	☐	
20. Return to Community Referral	☐	☐	

B. Signature of RN Coordinator for CAA Process and Date Signed

1. Signature
2. Date ☐☐ - ☐☐ - ☐☐☐☐
   Month   Day   Year

C. Signature of Person Completing Care Plan Decision and Date Signed

1. Signature
2. Date ☐☐ - ☐☐ - ☐☐☐☐
   Month   Day   Year

Finish the entire MDS before doing the CAAs

The nursing home staff should complete the entire resident assessment intrument and MDS before doing the CAAs. Some care areas need items from multiple sections to trigger.

Assessment of triggered care areas

CMS doesn't mandate any specific method for assessing triggered care areas. It does provide some of their recommended tools in Appendix C, but those are not required. It is the Quality Assessment and Assurance (QAA) Committee's responsibility to choose assessment tools that follow current clinical guidelines and be evidence-based or expert-endorsed.

V0100 (items from the most recent prior OBRA or scheduled PPS assessment)

If a resident has prior OBRA or scheduled PPS assessments since their most recent admission, including entry or re-entry, then the values from that assessment go in item V0100.

Section V	Care Area Assessment (CAA) Summary
V0100. Items From the Most Recent Prior OBRA or Scheduled PPS Assessment	
Complete only if A0310E = 0 and if the following is true for the **prior assessment**: A0310A = 01- 06 or A0310B = 01	
Enter Code	**A. Prior Assessment Federal OBRA Reason for Assessment** (A0310A value from prior assessment) 01. **Admission** assessment (required by day 14) 02. **Quarterly** review assessment 03. **Annual** assessment 04. **Significant change in status** assessment 05. **Significant correction** to **prior comprehensive** assessment 06. **Significant correction** to **prior quarterly** assessment 99. None of the above
Enter Code	**B. Prior Assessment PPS Reason for Assessment** (A0310B value from prior assessment) 01. **5-day** scheduled assessment 08. **IPA** - Interim Payment Assessment 99. None of the above
	C. Prior Assessment Reference Date (A2300 value from prior assessment) Month - Day - Year
Enter Score	**D. Prior Assessment Brief Interview for Mental Status (BIMS) Summary Score** (C0500 value from prior assessment)
Enter Score	**E. Prior Assessment Resident Mood Interview (PHQ-9©) Total Severity Score** (D0300 value from prior assessment)
Enter Score	**F. Prior Assessment Staff Assessment of Resident Mood (PHQ-9-OV) Total Severity Score** (D0600 value from prior assessment)

If V0100-A is 99 (none of the above), then the V0100-B must be 01 (5-day scheduled assessment) or 08 (IPA – interim payment assessment).

If V0100B is 99 (none of the above), then V0100A must be one of the items from 01 through 06, which are all OBRA assessments.

V0100A and V0100B cannot both be 99, which means that the values in the section are from neither an OBRA nor a PPS assessment.

Section X: Correction request

Section X is for identifying an MDS that will be modified or inactivated. You only have to do section X if:

- A0050 (type of record) = 2 (modify existing record)
- A0050 (type of record) = 3 (inactive existing record)

A0050. Type of Record	
Enter Code	1. **Add new record** → Continue to A0100, Facility Provider Numbers 2. **Modify existing record** → Continue to A0100, Facility Provider Numbers 3. **Inactivate existing record** → Skip to X0150, Type of Provider

Quality Improvement Evaluation System (QIES)

Nursing homes enter their MDS data into the **Quality Improvement Evaluation System** (**QIES**), which also includes the **Assessment Submission and Processing** (**ASAP**) system. The information that everyone enters is put into the national MDS database.

Information that is entered incorrectly into the MDS database

You can send modification requests to correct a QIES or ASAP record because of:

- transcription errors
- data entry errors
- software product errors,
- item coding errors
- other errors that require modification of the MDS database

Section X	Correction Request

Complete Section X only if A0050 = 2 or 3

Identification of Record to be Modified/Inactivated - The following items identify the existing assessment record that is in error. In this section, reproduce the information EXACTLY as it appeared on the existing erroneous record, even if the information is incorrect. This information is necessary to locate the existing record in the National MDS Database.

X0150. Type of Provider (A0200 on existing record to be modified/inactivated)

Enter Code ☐ Type of provider
1. **Nursing home (SNF/NF)**
2. **Swing Bed**

X0200. Name of Resident (A0500 on existing record to be modified/inactivated)

A. First name:
☐☐☐☐☐☐☐☐☐☐☐☐

C. Last name:
☐☐☐☐☐☐☐☐☐☐☐☐☐☐☐☐☐☐

X0300. Gender (A0800 on existing record to be modified/inactivated)

Enter Code ☐
1. **Male**
2. **Female**

X0400. Birth Date (A0900 on existing record to be modified/inactivated)

☐☐ - ☐☐ - ☐☐☐☐
Month   Day   Year

X0500. Social Security Number (A0600A on existing record to be modified/inactivated)

☐☐☐ - ☐☐ - ☐☐☐☐

X0570. Optional State Assessment (A0300A on existing record to be modified/inactivated)

Enter Code ☐ A. Is this assessment for state payment purposes only?
0. **No**
1. **Yes**

X0600. Type of Assessment (A0310 on existing record to be modified/inactivated)

Enter Code ☐☐ A. **Federal OBRA Reason for Assessment**
- 01. **Admission** assessment (required by day 14)
- 02. **Quarterly** review assessment
- 03. **Annual** assessment
- 04. **Significant change in status** assessment
- 05. **Significant correction** to **prior comprehensive** assessment
- 06. **Significant correction** to **prior quarterly** assessment
- 99. **None of the above**

Enter Code ☐☐ B. **PPS Assessment**
PPS Scheduled Assessment for a Medicare Part A Stay
- 01. **5-day** scheduled assessment

PPS Unscheduled Assessment for a Medicare Part A Stay
- 08. **IPA** - Interim Payment Assessment

Not PPS Assessment
- 99. **None of the above**

Enter Code ☐☐ F. **Entry/discharge reporting**
- 01. **Entry** tracking record
- 10. **Discharge** assessment-return not anticipated
- 11. **Discharge** assessment-return anticipated
- 12. **Death in facility** tracking record
- 99. **None of the above**

Enter Code ☐ H. **Is this a SNF Part A PPS Discharge Assessment?**
- 0. **No**
- 1. **Yes**

Section X	Correction Request

X0700. Date on existing record to be modified/inactivated - **Complete one only**

A. **Assessment Reference Date** (A2300 on existing record to be modified/inactivated) - Complete only if X0600F = 99

☐☐ - ☐☐ - ☐☐☐☐
Month   Day   Year

B. **Discharge Date** (A2000 on existing record to be modified/inactivated) - Complete only if X0600F = 10, 11, or 12

☐☐ - ☐☐ - ☐☐☐☐
Month   Day   Year

C. **Entry Date** (A1600 on existing record to be modified/inactivated) - Complete only if X0600F = 01

☐☐ - ☐☐ - ☐☐☐☐
Month   Day   Year

How to correct errors

There are two steps to fixing an error on a previous assessment.

1. In section X, write down the erroneous information from the existing record. This information is used to locate the existing record in the national MDS database.
2. Copy the information from original section A or the previous record to items X0200 through X0700.

    > For example, if a resident's birthday is February 15, 1929, but it was entered as March 15, 1929, then the erroneous date (02-15-1929) goes into X0400.

3. Fill in the number of corrections that you want to make to the new MDS

Item set code (ISC)

The item set code (ISC) determines item sets.

Notes: RFA stands for re-entry tracking form.

Nursing home item set code (ISC) reference table, part 1

Description	ISC	OBRA RFA (A0310-A)	PPS RFA (A0310-B)
Comprehensive	NC	01, 03, 04, 05	01, 99
Quarterly	NQ	02, 06	01, 99
PPS	NP	99	01
PPS (optional)	IPA	99	08
OBRA discharge	ND	99	99
Tracking	NT	99	99
Part A PPS discharge	NPE	99	99

Nursing home item set code (ISC) reference table, part 2

Description	ISC	Entry or discharge (A0310F)	Part A PPS discharge (A0310H)
Comprehensive	NC	10, 11, 99	0, 1
Quarterly	NQ	10, 11, 99	0, 1
PPS	NP	10, 11, 99	0, 1
PPS (optional)	IPA	99	0
OBRA discharge	ND	10, 11	0, 1
Tracking	NT	01, 12	0
Part A PPS discharge	NPE	99	1

A0310. Type of Assessment	
Enter Code	**A. Federal OBRA Reason for Assessment** 01. **Admission** assessment (required by day 14) 02. **Quarterly** review assessment 03. **Annual** assessment 04. **Significant change in status** assessment 05. **Significant correction** to **prior comprehensive** assessment 06. **Significant correction** to **prior quarterly** assessment 99. **None of the above**
Enter Code	**B. PPS Assessment** **PPS Scheduled Assessment for a Medicare Part A Stay** 01. **5-day** scheduled assessment **PPS Unscheduled Assessment for a Medicare Part A Stay** 08. **IPA** - Interim Payment Assessment **Not PPS Assessment** 99. **None of the above**
Enter Code	**E. Is this assessment the first assessment** (OBRA, Scheduled PPS, or Discharge) **since the most recent admission/entry or reentry?** 0. **No** 1. **Yes**
Enter Code	**F. Entry/discharge reporting** 01. **Entry** tracking record 10. **Discharge** assessment-**return not anticipated** 11. **Discharge** assessment-**return anticipated** 12. **Death in facility** tracking record 99. **None of the above**
Enter Code	**G. Type of discharge** - Complete only if A0310F = 10 or 11 1. **Planned** 2. **Unplanned**
Enter Code	**G1. Is this a SNF Part A Interrupted Stay?** 0. **No** 1. **Yes**
Enter Code	**H. Is this a SNF Part A PPS Discharge Assessment?** 0. **No** 1. **Yes**

These assessment items determine the item sets:

- A0310-A (federal OBRA reason for assessment)
- A0310-B (PPS assessment)
- A0310-F (Entry or discharge reporting)
- A0310-H (Is this a SNF Part A PPS discharge assessment?)

Changing assessment type

If the item set code doesn't change, then section A0310 (assessment type) can be modified.

For example, the admission assessment and a 5-day PPS assessment both have the same ISC code, which is NC. If a nurse first enters it into QIES as only an admission assessment, then she can later change it to admission assessment and 5-day PPS assessment.

However, the quarterly assessment and a significant change in status have different ISC codes. So, you can't modify the assessment type in this case.

Section Z: Assessment administration

Z0100. Medicare Part A Billing
A. Medicare Part A HIPPS code:
B. Version code:

Section Z is for billing information and the signatures of people who complete the assessment.

Z0100 (Medicare Part A billing)

Section Z0100 shows two codes:

- the **Patient Driven Payment Model** (**PDPM**) case mix version codes
- **Health Insurance Prospective Payment System** (**HIPPS**) modifier codes, which are based on the type of assessment done

PDPM will eventually replace the RUG system as a way of paying federal and state money to nursing homes. I don't understand PDPM myself. Hopefully one day I'll be able to learn PDPM and then write a book about it.

HIPPS is a five-position billing code for skilled nursing facilities (SNF). The first four positions represent the PDPM case mix code, and the fifth position is the assessment type indicator. The MDS software will usually automatically calculate what the HIPPS code is.

Z0400 (signatures of persons completing the assessment or entry/death reporting)

Attesting for accuracy: The person who selects the MDS item response is responsible for its accuracy. Everyone who completes a portion of the MDS has to sign at section Z0400, attest to the accuracy of the portion that they did, and list the items and sections they did and the date that they completed them.

Registered nurse not required to sign the Z0400 attestation: The RN assessment coordinator is not required to sign the Z0400 attestation. She only has to sign the portion of the MDS that she herself completed.

Section Z — Assessment Administration

Z0400. Signature of Persons Completing the Assessment or Entry/Death Reporting

I certify that the accompanying information accurately reflects resident assessment information for this resident and that I collected or coordinated collection of this information on the dates specified. To the best of my knowledge, this information was collected in accordance with applicable Medicare and Medicaid requirements. I understand that this information is used as a basis for ensuring that residents receive appropriate and quality care, and as a basis for payment from federal funds. I further understand that payment of such federal funds and continued participation in the government-funded health care programs is conditioned on the accuracy and truthfulness of this information, and that I may be personally subject to or may subject my organization to substantial criminal, civil, and/or administrative penalties for submitting false information. I also certify that I am authorized to submit this information by this facility on its behalf.

	Signature	Title	Sections	Date Section Completed
A.				
B.				
C.				
D.				
E.				
B.				
C.				
D.				
E.				
F.				
G.				
H.				
I.				
J.				
K.				
L.				

Z0500. Signature of RN Assessment Coordinator Verifying Assessment Completion

A. Signature:

B. Date RN Assessment Coordinator signed assessment as complete:

☐☐ - ☐☐ - ☐☐☐☐
Month   Day   Year

Date: The date in Z0400 is the day that a section was completed.

> **Date of completion, not day of signature**: The Z0400 is not for the date that someone signed a section. If a staff member can't sign on the day that a section was completed, then when she gets around to it, she should sign the day that the section was originally completed.
>
> **Multiple completion dates**: An assessor can sign with more than one date. People usually attach notes in the clinical record for when staff completed individual items, especially with interview questions. For example, if a nurse did the pain interview (section J) on Monday and then two items in functional status (section G) on Wednesday, then there would be one signature for section J on Monday and one signature for the two items section G on Wednesday.

Items with standard lookback periods and full observation periods: Some items on the assessment require observation of the resident throughout the entire lookback period. The Z0400 date for these items should be no earlier than the day after the ARD.

Items with non-standard lookback periods: Some items don't have a lookback period or have a non-standard lookback period. These items can be completed at various time during the completion process. For example, the resident's name and demographic information can be completed anytime. Meanwhile, resident interviews should be completed the day of the ARD or the day before the ARD.

Z0500 (signature of RN assessment coordinator verifying assessment completion)

Item **Z0500A** is for the RN assessment coordinator. This means that the assessment is complete. The signature of Z0500A does not attest to the accuracy of the MDS.

Z0500. Signature of RN Assessment Coordinator Verifying Assessment Completion	
A. Signature:	B. Date RN Assessment Coordinator signed assessment as complete: Month - Day - Year

The PPS and quarterly assessments do not require the CAA summary (section V).

Z0500. Signature of RN Assessment Coordinator Verifying Assessment Completion	
A. Signature:	B. Date RN Assessment Coordinator signed assessment as complete: ☐☐ - ☐☐ - ☐☐☐☐ Month　Day　Year

Item **Z0500-B** is the date that the RN assessment coordinator signed at Z0500-A (signature of RN assessment coordinator). This is the date of the original signature. If someone prints copies of this, then someone should write a note that the form is a copy of the original.

Wait until everyone is done: Because Z0500-A means that the entire MDS assessment is complete, the RN assessment coordinator shouldn't sign it until all the other staff members have finished completing their sections and have signed off on it.

Wait until after the ARD: The RN assessment coordinator shouldn't sign before the assessment reference date because the assessment can't end before the observation period ends.

A2300. Assessment Reference Date
Observation end date: ☐☐-☐☐-☐☐☐☐ Month Day Year

The assessment reference date (ARD) is in item A2300.

Z0500. Signature of RN Assessment Coordinator Verifying Assessment Completion	
A. Signature:	B. Date RN Assessment Coordinator signed assessment as complete: ☐☐-☐☐-☐☐☐☐ Month Day Year

Admission assessments must be completed with 14 days of admission.

Significant change of status assessment must be completed within 14 days of identification of a significant change in status.

Significant correction to prior assessments must be completed within 14 days of identification of a need for correction.

Comprehensive assessments must be completed by the CAA assessment process signature date (V0200-B). This is also the date of CAA completion.

For all other assessments, the date at Z0500-B has to be no later than 14 days after the assessment reference date (A2300).

www.ingramcontent.com/pod-product-compliance
Lightning Source LLC
Chambersburg PA
CBHW060419220526
45465CB00008B/2949